Cognitive Biases in Surgical Practice

Alvaro Sanabria · Carlos Betancourt

Cognitive Biases in Surgical Practice

Springer

Alvaro Sanabria
Head and Neck Section
Department of Surgery
School of Medicine
University of Antioquia
Medellín, Colombia

Carlos Betancourt
Head and Neck Section
Department of Surgery
School of Medicine
University of Antioquia
Medellín, Colombia

ISBN 978-3-032-20376-2 ISBN 978-3-032-20377-9 (eBook)
https://doi.org/10.1007/978-3-032-20377-9

The original submitted manuscript has been translated into English. The translation was done using artificial intelligence. A subsequent revision was performed by the author(s) to further refine the work and to ensure that the translation is appropriate concerning content and scientific correctness. It may, however, read stylistically different from a conventional translation.

This Springer imprint is published by the registered company Springer Nature Switzerland AG
The registered company address is: Gewerbestrasse 11, 6330 Cham, Switzerland

Preface

Understanding human behavior, motivations, and purposes has always been one of humanity's greatest aspirations. The implications of this knowledge are so vast that it would be impossible to summarize them in these pages. Suffice it to say that there is no facet of human life that is not impacted by the way people think, decide, and act. It is not surprising, then, that disciplines as diverse as philosophy, sociology, psychology, and economics have attempted to answer this question from different and, at times, even contradictory perspectives.

For decades, these approaches shared a common premise, the idea that human beings are rational agents, oriented toward maximizing benefits and minimizing losses. The emergence of the concept of cognitive biases decisively challenged this paradigm. Far from confirming a systematic rationality, this body of knowledge showed that human reasoning is profoundly fallible and that the brain is, under certain circumstances, predisposed to predictable errors in analysis and decision-making. This finding represented a conceptual turning point that forced a rethinking of the foundations of multiple disciplines, with consequences that extended to all areas of knowledge.

For the authors, understanding how these phenomena influence the practice of medicine and surgery, particularly in decision-making under conditions of uncertainty and pressure, has been a central interest. The search for answers has guided us to dedicate time to critical reading and reflection. However, despite the abundance of literature on cognitive biases in other fields, its concrete application to medical, and especially surgical, practice remains limited and fragmented.

This book is not intended to be an exhaustive treatise or a reference text that systematically covers all the cognitive biases described. Nor does it seek to replace specialized works in cognitive psychology, behavioral economics, or decision theory. Its purpose is more modest: to serve as a starting point that allows surgeons to become familiar with the topic and recognize how everyday problems and difficulties in surgical practice can be explained, at least in part, by the influence of cognitive biases.

To make a topic to which surgeons are not routinely exposed more accessible, we structured this book around real-life stories, drawn from clinical situations, formal and informal discussions before, during, and after surgical procedures, and shared experiences. This narrative approach allowed for a technical and rigorous, yet deliberately simple, style, avoiding unnecessary complexities and prioritizing a fluid, understandable, and engaging reading experience. We believe that clinical narratives are a powerful tool for linking abstract concepts with the concrete reality of surgical decision-making.

Our intention is not only to describe how cognitive biases operate in routine decisions but also to offer readers conceptual tools that allow them to identify and recognize these biases and to reflect on strategies for mitigating their potentially harmful effects or, in certain contexts, directing them to benefit patients' interests and safety.

We acknowledge that, in some cases, the concepts presented may involve simplifications. These are due to the introductory nature of the work and the explicit intention of facilitating a first approach to the topic. We hope that this book will stimulate curiosity, generate questions, and motivate the reader to reach more complex theoretical and empirical approaches. If, upon finishing the book, the surgeon recognizes themselves in the stories narrated and feels compelled to explore the study of cognitive biases in greater depth, we will have achieved the objective of this work.

Medellín, Colombia

Alvaro Sanabria
Carlos Betancourt

Acknowledgments

This book would not have been possible without the constant and generous support of my family. I wish to express, first and foremost, my deepest gratitude to my wife, Martha, and my children, Álvaro José and Martha Lucía, for being my unwavering support in every project I have undertaken. Their understanding, patience, and companionship have allowed me to dedicate much of the time that rightfully belongs to them to these intellectual pursuits. To them I owe not only daily encouragement but also the balance and serenity necessary to persevere.

My gratitude also extends to my parents, Álvaro and Consuelo Inés, who instilled in me from an early age a love for science, stimulated my intellectual curiosity, and never ceased to believe in my potential to become who I am today. Their example, trust, and unconditional support have been a constant guide throughout my personal and professional life.

–Alvaro Sanabria

This book would never have come to life without the love, support, and generosity of so many people to whom I am deeply grateful:

Above all, I thank God for the gift of life and for the talents, strength, and opportunities He has placed in my path.

My gratitude also goes to my parents, Carlos and Rosario, my greatest encouragers throughout my life. And to you, Dad, thank you especially for your invaluable help, guidance, and dedication in reviewing and refining this book.

To my beloved wife, Oli, thank you for your unconditional love, patience, and sacrifices. Your willingness to carry so many responsibilities so that I could devote myself fully to this project made this dream possible.

And finally, to my precious daughters, Arantza and Avril: thank you for giving up moments that belonged to you so that I could pursue this dream. Your smiles, your love, and your presence are my greatest inspiration and all I need to be truly happy.

–Carlos Betancourt

Contents

About the Authors

Alvaro Sanabria Medical Doctor and Surgeon, National University of Colombia. Bogota, Colombia. Specialist in General Surgery, University of Antioquia, Medellín, Colombia. Specialist in Head and Neck Surgery, AC Camargo Hospital, São Paulo, Brazil. Fellowship in Microsurgical Reconstruction, Autonomous University of Barcelona, Spain. Master of Science in Clinical Epidemiology, Pontificia Universidad Javeriana, Bogotá, Colombia. Master of Science in Health and Pharmaceutical Economics, Pompeu Fabra University, Barcelona, Spain. Master of Science in Behavioral Studies, EAFIT University, Medellín, Colombia. Doctor in Oncology, Celestino Burroul School of Cancerology, São Paulo, Brazil. He currently holds the position of Full Professor in the Department of Surgery at the University of Antioquia, Medellín, Colombia. He serves as the Coordinator of the Head and Neck Surgery Fellowship and practices as a head and neck surgeon at San Vicente Fundación University Hospital, Clinica Las Vegas-Quirón Salud Group, and Clinica Somer, Colombia.

Carlos Betancourt Medical Doctor and Surgeon, UCLA, Barquisimeto, Venezuela. Specialist in General Surgery, UCLA, Barquisimeto, Venezuela. Specialist in Head and Neck Surgery, Hospital das Clinicas, University of São Paulo, São Paulo, Brazil. He currently holds the position of Professor in the Department of Surgery at the University of Antioquia, Medellín, Colombia. He practices as a head and neck surgeon at San Vicente Fundación University Hospital, Clinica Las Vegas-Quirón Salud Group, and Alma Mater Hospital of Antioquia, Colombia.

List of Figures

Chapter 1
Introduction

On October 9, 2002, the world witnessed an unprecedented event. For the first time, a non-economist was awarded the Nobel Prize in Economics. The recipient, Daniel Kahneman, a trained psychologist, earned the prize for his work integrating cognitive psychology into economic sciences, particularly regarding human reasoning and decision-making under uncertainty. His research, initiated 30 years earlier in collaboration with Amos Tversky, revolutionized the field of psychology and laid the foundation for what would later become a new discipline known as Behavioral Economics. (Lewis, 2016) His findings were so significant that they forever changed the central model of traditional economics. Before Kahneman and Tversky, this model was based on the belief that humans are perfectly rational agents, capable of processing all available information, evaluating every option, and making the best decision to maximize their own utility (*homo economicus*). Kahneman applied his discoveries in cognitive psychology to the decision-making process, demonstrating that this traditional model did not describe real-world human behavior. His work made it possible to recognize and understand that human decisions are systematically influenced by psychological factors (heuristics and biases) that elude any logical reasoning. (Kahneman, 2011) Fifteen years later, Richard Thaler, an unconventional economist from the University of Chicago's School of Economics, who worked closely with Kahneman, was awarded the Nobel Prize in Economics by the Swedish National Bank for constructing the theoretical framework that connects Kahneman's psychological findings with formal economic analysis (Thaler, 2015).

Thus, with Kahneman, Tversky, and Thaler, Behavioral Economics, a field dedicated to studying how human decisions systematically and predictably deviate from rationality under the influence of heuristics and cognitive biases, was born. The impact and scope of their research quickly extended beyond the economic sphere. When applied to personal finance and marketing, it enabled a better understanding of why investors behave erratically (for example, why they hold on to losing stocks instead of selling them) and why certain advertising campaigns are more effective when they appeal to specific emotions (such as when a time limit is set on promotions).

A. Sanabria and C. Betancourt, *Cognitive Biases in Surgical Practice*,
https://doi.org/10.1007/978-3-032-20377-9_1

In public policy, it led to the development of interventions that influence people's decisions for their own benefit without restricting their options (for example, encouraging personal savings or organ donation through choice architecture) (Thaler & Sunstein, 2009).

Therefore, there is no area or field that escapes the evaluation of human behavior and the way decisions are made. Advertising, finance, politics, the administration of justice, management, and so on, have all been profoundly influenced by the innovative concepts of this new discipline. Moreover, amid the "*irrationality*" of human behavior, Behavioral Economics makes it largely possible to anticipate the direction of such behavior. By understanding the most prevalent heuristics and cognitive biases in specific scenarios, it is possible to predict how individuals will behave and the decisions they are likely to make.

Medicine is no exception. However, unlike the areas mentioned above, little research has been conducted or written about how heuristics and cognitive biases influence physicians' professional practice and their interactions with patients. (Howard, 2018) Most of the available information has focused on assessing the prevalence of the most common biases, and few studies have attempted to explain their impact on physicians' professional activities or what can be done to mitigate their harmful effects.

While there is very little available in medicine, in the more specific field of surgery, there is virtually nothing. This text therefore emerges as an attempt to address these questions. Within it, the reader will find clear explanations of the cognitive biases that, in the authors' opinion, have the greatest impact on the professional practice of surgeons. Similarly, at the end of each chapter, a series of strategies to mitigate their effects is provided.

It is important to acknowledge that, as with any retrospective analysis, the examples discussed may themselves be subject to the cognitive biases under examination. The risk of an "*illusion of understanding*" is real and may lead to misinterpretation. To mitigate this, we have deliberately selected illustrative cases in which the influence of a specific bias appears particularly salient, potentially serving as a primary explanatory factor. Notably, empirical data on the impact of cognitive biases in surgical decision-making remain limited. Additionally, assigning a particular bias to a clinical narrative is inherently subjective. Readers may interpret a given scenario through the lens of a different bias than the one proposed. While we remain mindful of these limitations, the purpose of each case is to explore the possible consequences of a specific bias, acknowledging that every decision is likely shaped by multiple interacting cognitive influences.

The book has been structured so that each chapter functions as an independent unit, allowing it to be read either in the sequence designed by the authors or by jumping directly to the chapters of greatest interest. In the appendix, a set of checklists has been developed, which can be used in the various scenarios faced by surgeons as a strategy to mitigate the effects of biases. We hope that this proposal will be useful and help shed light on this little-studied topic, which is of critical importance for surgical decision-making.

References

Howard, J. (2018). *Cognitive Errors and Diagnostic Mistakes: A Case-Based Guide to Critical Thinking in Medicine.* Springer International Publishing.

Kahneman, D. (2011). *Thinking, Fast and Slow*. Penguin Books Limited.

Lewis, M. (2016). *The Undoing Project: A Friendship that Changed the World*. Penguin Books Limited.

Thaler, R. H. (2015). *Misbehaving: The Making of Behavioral Economics*. W. W. Norton.

Thaler, R. H., & Sunstein, C. R. (2009). *Nudge: Improving Decisions About Health, Wealth, and Happiness*. Penguin Publishing Group.

Chapter 2
Cognitive Biases: History and Definition

The Theory of Dual-Process Thinking

Long before the seminal studies of Kahneman and Tversky in the 1970s, several researchers were already questioning the idea that people always make logical decisions. In the mid-twentieth century, George Katona and Herbert Simon conducted studies on cognitive limitations and behavioral anomalies. Katona, who studied Gestalt psychology, identified how individuals' expectations and subjective attitudes influence their behavior, assessing how consumers make judgments that do not always follow logical reasoning. Meanwhile, Simon proposed the concept of "*bounded rationality,* "which holds that people constantly seek quick and efficient answers due to the limitations of their thinking. (Svornenčík & Truc, 2022) These early efforts challenged the notion of the fully rational human being and enabled a different understanding of decision-making. Their observations, initially overlooked, would later prove crucial for the formalization of cognitive bias theory.

The formalization of dual-process theory of thought became popular in the 1970s and 1980s, following the contributions of Daniel Kahneman and Amos Tversky. In their seminal article " *Judgment under Uncertainty: Heuristics and Biases* " (Tversky & Kahneman, 1974), they laid the groundwork for the theory by describing two types of thinking: System 1, which is fast, automatic, and intuitive, and System 2, which is slow, deliberative, and analytical. For the first time, cognitive patterns and their errors were systematically studied, demonstrating that people make decisions that are not based on logic, a formulation entirely opposed to the prevailing idea of rational and calculating *homo economicus.* (Yamagishi et al., 2014) This had described individuals as agents who act to maximize their well-being given the constraints they face, and which was widely used in economics and the social sciences through **rational choice theory.** (Green, 2002).

Kahneman's advances ultimately earned him the Nobel Prize in Economics in 2002. (Rabin, 2003) Kahneman's renowned 2011 book, " *Thinking, Fast and Slow* " (Kahneman, 2012), explored these ideas in greater depth. Subsequently, Keith

A. Sanabria and C. Betancourt, *Cognitive Biases in Surgical Practice*,
https://doi.org/10.1007/978-3-032-20377-9_2

Stanovich (Stanovich, 1999) and Jonathan Evans (Evans, 2003) contributed to the theory by examining the details of how these two systems interact and influence decision-making in different situations.

The dual-process theory was fundamental in the development of Behavioral Economics, providing a psychological and conceptual foundation to explain why real-world decision-making often deviates from conventional economic models. Behavioral economists, building on the findings of Kahneman and Tversky, recognized that numerous decisions are influenced by the intuitive and rapid thinking of System 1. This idea, clearly reflected in the psychological and intellectual journey narrated in *The Undoing Project* (Lewis, 2016), gives support to Richard Thaler's work in *Misbehaving* (Thaler, 2015). Thaler demonstrated that systematic deviations from rationality, such as loss aversion, mental accounting, and the status quo bias, could be anticipated and elucidated through the interaction of these two cognitive systems. The incorporation of psychological realism into economic theory fundamentally transformed the understanding of human behavior across all domains, especially in finance, medicine, and public policy.

Heuristics and Cognitive Biases

Heuristics are mental tools or general rules used by individuals to facilitate decision-making and problem-solving. People can quickly judge and decide what to do with limited information by using these mental tools. There are several reasons supporting their use. Heuristics help individuals make rapid decisions while keeping their mental resources available (**cognitive speed**), (Gigerenzer & Gaissmaier, 2011) reduce the amount of thinking required to solve a problem (**cognitive load, processing efficiency**), (Tversky & Kahneman, 1974) enable quick action in situations with limited information (**adaptation to uncertainty**), (Gigerenzer & Goldstein, 1996) aid survival in environments where rapid decisions are crucial (**evolutionary adaptation**) (Gigerenzer et al., 2012), and provide emotional support for the decision (**satisfaction effect**). (Simon, 1956).

In medicine, some examples of heuristics include:

1. Availability of information: (Elston, 2020) The surgeon estimates the frequency of a disease by recalling recent cases that are easy to remember. Example: The rule that rare diseases come in pairs, used to explain situations where a patient with an uncommon condition is seen within a short period, and soon after, another similar case is encountered.
2. Representativeness: (Richie & Josephson, 2018) The surgeon adjusts a diagnosis because the symptoms resemble those of another condition considered representative. Example: The use of a diagnostic triad (Beck's triad in cardiac tamponade).
3. Anchoring-and-adjustment: (Armstrong et al., 2023) The surgeon is influenced by their initial opinion or impression (the "anchor"). Example: A female patient

with right lower quadrant abdominal pain in the middle of the menstrual cycle leading to the exclusion of acute appendicitis.
4. Recognition: (Greul et al., 2023) The surgeon may favor a diagnosis or treatment with which they are more familiar due to greater knowledge. Example: Choosing a first-generation cephalosporin for a pleural infection because they are more familiar with it than with second-generation cephalosporins.
5. Satisfaction of search: (Huynh et al., 2021) The surgeon identifies an abnormality on an image and stops searching for other abnormalities. Example: During follow-up for colon cancer, a single pulmonary nodule is found on a chest CT and is assumed to be a metastasis.
6. Diagnostic momentum: (Webster et al., 2021) A surgeon makes a diagnosis in the morning, and those reviewing the patient later in the day accept it without further discussion. Example: The patient presents with psychomotor agitation and is considered to have delirium. No one reconsiders the diagnosis of delirium.

In contrast, cognitive biases are systematic deviations in thought processes that occur when individuals make decisions without relying on logic or objective evidence. These errors arise from the use of mental shortcuts (heuristics) or from perceptual flaws that alter the way information is processed, leading to incorrect decisions. Similar to heuristics, cognitive biases are mental tools that facilitate the understanding of a complex reality and reduce cognitive load (Tversky & Kahneman, 1974); they help improve decision-making under uncertainty (Haselton et al., 2009), increase the speed of information processing (Kahneman, 2012), assist in coping with emotionally challenging situations (Taylor & Brown, 1988), and support communication and collaboration (Mercier & Sperber, 2011); however, they often result in poor decision-making.

Some examples of cognitive biases in medicine include:

1. **Confirmation** bias: (Elston, 2020) The surgeon only considers information that supports a diagnosis they have already made and ignores evidence that contradicts it. Example: The surgeon believes the patient has pancreatitis due to elevated amylase, but disregards the normal lipase value.
2. **Overconfidence** bias: (Bushuven et al., 2019) The surgeon is overly confident in their ability to manage a patient and does not seek assistance. Example: In the midst of a traumatic pancreatoduodenal surgery, the surgeon believes they can perform an emergency Whipple procedure instead of opting for damage control.
3. **Sunk cost** bias: (Elston, 2022) The surgeon has invested time, money, and effort in a treatment plan but refuses to abandon it, even when there is evidence it is not working. Example: The surgeon observes signs of ischemia in a microvascular flap but decides to continue monitoring instead of reoperating.
4. **Hindsight** bias: (Dawson et al., 1988) The surgeon believes that an event that has occurred can be clearly explained by a previous intervention, which seems obvious in retrospect. Example: Faced with an intestinal fistula, the surgeon concludes it was due to a technical error that was not initially recognized.
5. **Bandwagon** bias: (Mailoo, 2015) The surgeon holds an opinion on a matter, but because it differs from the majority view, chooses not to express or defend

it. Example: In a board meeting, the surgeon believes observation is best for a patient, but the group prefers surgery, so the surgeon remains silent and the patient undergoes unnecessary surgery.

6. **Fundamental attribution** error: (Croskerry et al., 2008) The surgeon attributes others' actions to intrinsic factors and their own to extrinsic factors. Example: The surgeon criticizes a colleague for not following guideline recommendations but justifies their own noncompliance due to the "particularities" of the case.

Heuristics and cognitive biases are two different, yet interconnected, forms of decision-making and judgment. Heuristics are useful shortcuts for navigating a complex world, as they help us find quick answers by relying on easily accessible knowledge. However, excessive reliance on these shortcuts can lead to systematic errors in the thinking process, which alter the way we perceive and respond to the world. In most cases, these cognitive biases result in poor decision-making. (Kahneman & Tversky, 1973).

References

Armstrong, B. A., Dutescu, I. A., Tung, A., Carter, D. N., Trbovich, P. L., Wong, S., Saposnik, G., & Grantcharov, T. (2023). Cognitive biases in surgery: Systematic review. *The British Journal of Surgery, 110*(6), 645–654. https://doi.org/10.1093/bjs/znad004

Bushuven, S., Weidenbusch, M., Mohr, S., Delis, A., Fischer, M. R., Juenger, J., & Dettenkofer, M. (2019). Cognitive bias in professional hand hygiene and feedback: A national online survey on overconfidence in Germany. *Infection Control and Hospital Epidemiology, 40*(8), 943–946. https://doi.org/10.1017/ice.2019.156

Croskerry, P., Abbass, A. A., & Wu, A. W. (2008). How doctors feel: Affective issues in patient safety. *The Lancet, 372*(9645), 1205–1206.

Dawson, N. V., Arkes, H. R., Siciliano, C., Blinkhorn, R., Lakshmanan, M., & Petrelli, M. (1988). Hindsight bias: An impediment to accurate probability estimation in clinicopathologic conferences. *Medical Decision Making, 8*(4), 259–264. https://doi.org/10.1177/0272989x8800800406

Elston, D. M. (2020). Confirmation bias in medical decision-making. *Journal of the American Academy of Dermatology, 82*(3), 572. https://doi.org/10.1016/j.jaad.2019.06.1286

Elston, D. M. (2022). Sunk cost bias. *Journal of the American Academy of Dermatology, 86*(3), 527. https://doi.org/10.1016/j.jaad.2019.09.027

Evans, J. S. B. (2003). In two minds: Dual-process accounts of reasoning. *Trends in Cognitive Sciences, 7*(10), 454–459.

Gigerenzer, G., & Gaissmaier, W. (2011). Heuristic decision making. *Annual Review of Psychology, 62*, 451–482.

Gigerenzer, G., & Goldstein, D. G. (1996). Reasoning the fast and frugal way: Models of bounded rationality. *Psychological Review, 103*(4), 650.

Gigerenzer, G., Todd, P. M., & Group, A. R. Group, A. R. (2012). Ecological rationality: Intelligence in the world. Oxford University Press.

Green, S. L. (2002). Rational choice theory: An overview. In *Baylor University Faculty development seminar on rational choice theory* (pp. 1–72). Baylor University.

Greul, A., Schweisfurth, T. G., & Raasch, C. (2023). Does familiarity with an idea bias its evaluation? *PLoS One, 18*(7), e0286968. https://doi.org/10.1371/journal.pone.0286968

Haselton, M. G., Bryant, G. A., Wilke, A., Frederick, D. A., Galperin, A., Frankenhuis, W. E., & Moore, T. (2009). Adaptive rationality: An evolutionary perspective on cognitive bias. *Social Cognition, 27*(5), 733–763.

Huynh, J. D., Rhodes, S. C., Hatton, J. F., & Khademi, J. A. (2021). Satisfaction of search in periapical radiograph interpretation. *Journal of Endodontics, 47*(2), 291–296. https://doi.org/10.1016/j.joen.2020.11.001

Kahneman, D. (2012). Thinking, fast and slow. *Debate.*

Kahneman, D., & Tversky, A. (1973). On the psychology of prediction. *Psychological Review, 80*(4), 237.

Lewis, M. (2016). *The undoing project: A friendship that changed the world*. Penguin Books Limited.

Mailoo, V. (2015). Common sense or cognitive bias and groupthink: Does it belong in our clinical reasoning? *The British Journal of General Practice, 65*(630), 27. https://doi.org/10.3399/bjgp15X683173

Mercier, H., & Sperber, D. (2011). Why do humans reason? Arguments for an argumentative theory. *Behavioral and Brain Sciences, 34*(2), 57–74.

Rabin, M. (2003). The Nobel memorial prize for Daniel Kahneman. *The Scandinavian Journal of Economics, 105*(2), 157–180. http://www.jstor.org/stable/3441039

Richie, M., & Josephson, S. A. (2018). Quantifying heuristic bias: Anchoring, availability, and representativeness. *Teaching and Learning in Medicine, 30*(1), 67–75. https://doi.org/10.1080/10401334.2017.1332631

Simon, H. A. (1956). Rational choice and the structure of the environment. *Psychological Review, 63*(2), 129.

Stanovich, K. E. (1999). *Who is rational?: Studies of individual differences in reasoning*. Psychology Press.

Svorenčík, A., & Truc, A. (2022). *A history of behavioral economics and its applications: What we know and future research directions.* https://napnationalacademies.org/resource/26874/BE_history_20221009.pdf

Taylor, S. E., & Brown, J. D. (1988). Illusion and Well-being: A social psychological perspective on mental health. *Psychological Bulletin, 103*(2), 193.

Thaler, R. H. (2015). *Misbehaving: The making of behavioral economics*. Norton.

Tversky, A., & Kahneman, D. (1974). Judgment under uncertainty: Heuristics and biases. *Science, 185*(4157), 1124–1131. https://doi.org/doi:10.1126/science.185.4157.1124

Webster, C. S., Taylor, S., & Weller, J. M. (2021). Cognitive biases in diagnosis and decision making during anesthesia and intensive care. *BJA Educ, 21*(11), 420–425. https://doi.org/10.1016/j.bjae.2021.07.004

Yamagishi, T., Li, Y., Takagishi, H., Matsumoto, Y., & Kiyonari, T. (2014). In search of Homo economicus. *Psychological Science, 25*(9), 1699–1711. https://doi.org/10.1177/0956797614538065

Chapter 3
Impact of Cognitive Biases on Clinical Practice

In the complex world of clinical and surgical professional practice, the application of dual-process theory has become a fundamental framework for understanding how physicians make decisions. According to this theory (Kahneman, 2012), thought processes are shaped by two distinct brain systems. System 1, which is simple and automatic, operates quickly and efficiently by relying on shortcuts and rapid decisions; however, it can introduce biases that affect how patients are diagnosed and treated. For example, if a physician encounters a patient with common symptoms similar to those of the flu, they may quickly make that diagnosis due to familiarity with the illness, even though it may not necessarily be correct. System 2, on the other hand, engages in a more reflective process that requires concentration, logic, critical thinking, and effort. When applied in medicine, this system is particularly useful for verifying or correcting the rapid decisions made by System 1. In the same example, a physician might use System 2 to consider the differential diagnoses for this apparently flu-like presentation, which would help them obtain a more comprehensive understanding of the patient's condition.

When making any decision, including clinical ones, the metaphor of the elephant and the rider is often used (Haidt, 2019). System 1, the intuitive and impulsive part of thinking, is like an *elephant* that moves first, as it is naturally sensitive to the details of the patient's context and represents the surgeon's visceral component, allowing real-time decisions based on years of experience and rapid judgments. At the same time, System 2, the *rider,* is the part that thinks, analyzes, and tries to understand why the elephant acts irrationally, serving as the reflective and conscious element that intervenes to find logical reasons to explain the elephant's automatic actions.

A. Sanabria and C. Betancourt, *Cognitive Biases in Surgical Practice*,
https://doi.org/10.1007/978-3-032-20377-9_3

Effect of Cognitive Biases on the Practice of Medicine and Surgery

When biases are not detected and controlled, they can lead to incorrect diagnoses, inappropriate treatments, and suboptimal outcomes. Some studies indicate that approximately 90% of medical decisions may be influenced by cognitive biases (Blumenthal-Barby & Krieger, 2015; Watari et al., 2022), and even the most experienced physicians are susceptible to them.

Several cognitive biases have a significant impact in medical settings. Overconfidence, for example, strongly influences decision-making and can lead to inappropriate or unnecessary interventions. Availability bias may overestimate the danger associated with rare diseases by up to tenfold (McNeil et al., 1982). Anchoring bias can affect risk estimates by as much as 50% (Tversky & Kahneman, 1974). Confirmation bias accounts for up to 30% of diagnostic errors due to the lack of a more critical thought process (Nickerson, 1998). Loss aversion may prevent the offering of potentially beneficial but risky procedures, and the bandwagon effect influences the allocation of resources toward therapies that are popular but less effective (Waters et al., 2007).

In the exclusively surgical field, recent studies have shown that cognitive biases are common in decision-making and can have a significant impact on patient outcomes. Armstrong et al. (Armstrong et al., 2023) described several biases that significantly affect surgeons. Among these are anchoring bias, in which initial diagnostic impressions disproportionately influence subsequent decisions; availability bias, which distorts risk assessment based on recent or vivid cases; and confirmation bias, which leads physicians to prioritize information that supports their preexisting beliefs at the expense of other equally important data. Additionally, overconfidence and commission bias can affect individuals, especially in high-risk situations. In similar studies, MacDermid et al. (MacDermid et al., 2017) found that colorectal surgeons often rely on personal judgment and risk tolerance, rather than objective facts, when determining the need for a stoma following anterior rectal resection. Likewise, Whyte et al. (Whyte et al., 2022) found that surgeons, nurses, and patients were subject to similar cognitive biases, such as framing effects, confirmation bias, and illusion of control, when making decisions about elective breast reconstruction.

The consistency of these biases across various specialties and levels of experience indicates that they are not alleviated solely by skill, and may be deeply rooted in the cognitive mechanisms that influence surgical decision-making. Furthermore, they are often exacerbated by stress, the hierarchical structure of the profession, and emotionally charged circumstances.

Cognitive biases have consequences for patient safety and outcomes. Research shows that biases such as overconfidence, anchoring, and underestimation of the risk of complications can lead to errors or misguided decisions that could have been avoided (MacDermid et al., 2017). Similarly, Antonacci et al. (Antonacci et al., 2021) reported that cognitive errors were a major cause of intraoperative complications, and that biases during the diagnostic process and subsequent decision-making were often responsible.

On the other hand, decisions made in multidisciplinary meetings or decision boards are also susceptible to various cognitive biases that can affect clinical judgment. These settings are prone to authority bias, which occurs when individuals refrain from expressing their opinions out of deference to high-ranking figures; confirmation bias, which arises when individuals interpret data to support their preexisting beliefs; and the illusion of agreement, which occurs when individuals assume that silence implies support, thereby reinforcing group thinking. (Daily et al., 2025) Furthermore, in such environments, the need to make rapid decisions can facilitate the effects of availability bias, outcome bias, and loss aversion, especially when there is a history of recent or emotionally devastating cases. Moreover, when reputational consequences and public pressure are particularly intense, the impact of these biases becomes even greater.

The Importance of Awareness

Recognizing that biases exist and have a significant effect on clinical decision-making is the first step toward reducing their influence and impact. (Reilly et al., 2013) Awareness of these biases helps to seek evidence of their influence and to question initial impressions. Furthermore, it serves as a tool to prevent their entrenchment and persistence within the surgical community. (Karnick et al., 2021) Additionally, being aware of one's own thought processes (metacognition) enables the development of reflective thinking, facilitating the examination of decisions and the detection of potential biases.

Finally, adopting a mindset of continuous learning and growth encourages openness to feedback, facilitates collaboration and discussion, and supports the implementation of evidence-based practices. Several studies, such as that by Royce et al., assert that explicit education on cognitive biases during medical training has the potential to minimize diagnostic errors and improve patient safety (Royce et al., 2019). Similarly, a curriculum focused on diagnostic errors and cognitive biases increased the recognition of these issues among internal medicine residents (Reilly et al., 2013). However, Sherbino et al. were unable to reduce diagnostic errors among medical students when educational methods based on clinical reasoning and cognitive reinforcement techniques were used (Sherbino et al., 2014).

References

Antonacci, A. C., Dechario, S. P., Antonacci, C., Husk, G., Patel, V., Nicastro, J., Coppa, G., & Jarrett, M. (2021). Cognitive bias impact on Management of Postoperative Complications, medical error, and standard of care. *The Journal of Surgical Research, 258*, 47–53. https://doi.org/10.1016/j.jss.2020.08.040

Armstrong, B. A., Dutescu, I. A., Tung, A., Carter, D. N., Trbovich, P. L., Wong, S., Saposnik, G., & Grantcharov, T. (2023). Cognitive biases in surgery: Systematic review. *The British Journal of Surgery, 110*(6), 645–654. https://doi.org/10.1093/bjs/znad004

Blumenthal-Barby, J. S., & Krieger, H. (2015). Cognitive biases and heuristics in medical decision making: A critical review using a systematic search strategy. *Medical Decision Making, 35*(4), 539–557. https://doi.org/10.1177/0272989X14547740

Daily, J. A., Dalby, S., & Greiten, L. (2025). Cognitive biases in high-stakes decision-making: Implications for joint pediatric cardiology and cardiothoracic surgery conference. *Pediatric Cardiology, 46*(3), 536–543. https://doi.org/10.1007/s00246-024-03462-4

Haidt, J. (2019). *The righteous mind*. Editorial Planeta.

Kahneman, D. (2012). Thinking, fast and slow. *Debate.*

Karnick, A., Limberg, J., Bagautdinov, I., Stefanova, D., Aveson, V., Thiesmeyer, J., Fehling, D., & Fahey, T. J., 3rd. (2021). Can general surgery interns accurately assess their own technical skills? Analysis of cognitive bias in surgical residents' self-assessments. *Surgery, 170*(5), 1353–1358. https://doi.org/10.1016/j.surg.2021.04.008

MacDermid, E., Young, C. J., Moug, S. J., Anderson, R. G., & Shepherd, H. L. (2017). Heuristics and bias in rectal surgery. *International Journal of Colorectal Disease, 32*(8), 1109–1115. https://doi.org/10.1007/s00384-017-2823-7

McNeil, B. J., Pauker, S. G., Sox, H. C., Jr., & Tversky, A. (1982). On the elicitation of preferences for alternative therapies. *The New England Journal of Medicine, 306*(21), 1259–1262. https://doi.org/10.1056/NEJM198205273062103

Nickerson, R. S. (1998). Confirmation bias: A ubiquitous phenomenon in many guises. *Review of General Psychology, 2*(2), 175–220.

Reilly, J. B., Ogdie, A. R., Von Feldt, J. M., & Myers, J. S. (2013). Teaching about how doctors think: A longitudinal curriculum in cognitive bias and diagnostic error for residents. *BMJ Quality and Safety, 22*(12), 1044–1050. https://doi.org/10.1136/bmjqs-2013-001987

Royce, C. S., Hayes, M. M., & Schwartzstein, R. M. (2019). Teaching critical thinking: A case for instruction in cognitive biases to reduce diagnostic errors and improve patient safety. *Academic Medicine, 94*(2), 187–194. https://doi.org/10.1097/ACM.0000000000002518

Sherbino, J., Kulasegaram, K., Howey, E., & Norman, G. (2014). Ineffectiveness of cognitive forcing strategies to reduce biases in diagnostic reasoning: A controlled trial. *CJEM, 16*(1), 34–40. https://doi.org/10.2310/8000.2013.130860

Tversky, A., & Kahneman, D. (1974). Judgment under uncertainty: Heuristics and biases. *Science, 185*(4157), 1124–1131. https://doi.org/10.1126/science.185.4157.1124

Watari, T., Tokuda, Y., Amano, Y., Onigata, K., & Kanda, H. (2022). Cognitive bias and diagnostic errors among physicians in Japan: A self-reflection survey. *International Journal of Environmental Research and Public Health, 19*(8). https://doi.org/10.3390/ijerph19084645

Waters, E. A., Weinstein, N. D., Colditz, G. A., & Emmons, K. M. (2007). Reducing aversion to side effects in preventive medical treatment decisions. *Journal of Experimental Psychology: Applied, 13*(1), 11.

Whyte, S., Bray, L., Chan, H. F., Chan, R. J., Hunt, J., Peltz, T. S., Dulleck, U., & Hutmacher, D. W. (2022). Cognitive bias and therapy choice in breast reconstruction surgery decision-making. *Plastic and Reconstructive Surgery, 149*(4), 629e–637e. https://doi.org/10.1097/PRS.0000000000008903

Chapter 4
Hindsight Bias. The Death of James Garfield

The Problem

On November 2, 1880, James A. Garfield (Fig. 4.1) became the twentieth President of the United States of America. His rise to office, from his unexpected nomination as a candidate to his victory in the election, remains one of the greatest surprises in American political history. His legacy, however, would forever change many things, and not only in American politics.

Born into the deepest poverty in Orange, a rural area in northeastern Ohio in 1831, he lost his father at just 18 months old, which only worsened his already precarious situation. Through the great efforts of his mother and older brother, he studied at the Western Reserve Eclectic Institute from 1851 to 1854, during which time he also worked as a janitor at the same institution to help pay for his education. He quickly stood out as an excellent student, with an insatiable thirst for knowledge, which earned him an opportunity to study at Williams College in Massachusetts, where he graduated in 1856. He returned to the Eclectic Institute, where he taught mathematics, literature, and ancient languages, and became the college's principal in 1857, gaining visibility and some recognition in the region. At the same time, he studied law independently and was admitted to the Ohio bar in 1860 (Peskin, 1978).

Two factors would intertwine to force him to abandon his academic life: politics and war. In 1859, following the death of a state congressman, members of the Republican Party asked him to take the congressman's place in the upcoming election, which he would win by a wide margin two months later, thus beginning a career that would eventually lead him to the White House. However, just over a year after embarking on his political life, the American Civil War broke out. Garfield, a staunch abolitionist and advocate for equal rights for all people, quickly joined the Union Army, recruiting soldiers in his native region of Ohio, primarily among his former colleagues and students from the Eclectic Institute. By 1861, he was appointed colonel, and his men became the 42nd Regiment of the Union Army. After a few initial skirmishes, in mid-1861 he was assigned the mission of reclaiming the state of

A. Sanabria and C. Betancourt, *Cognitive Biases in Surgical Practice*,
https://doi.org/10.1007/978-3-032-20377-9_4

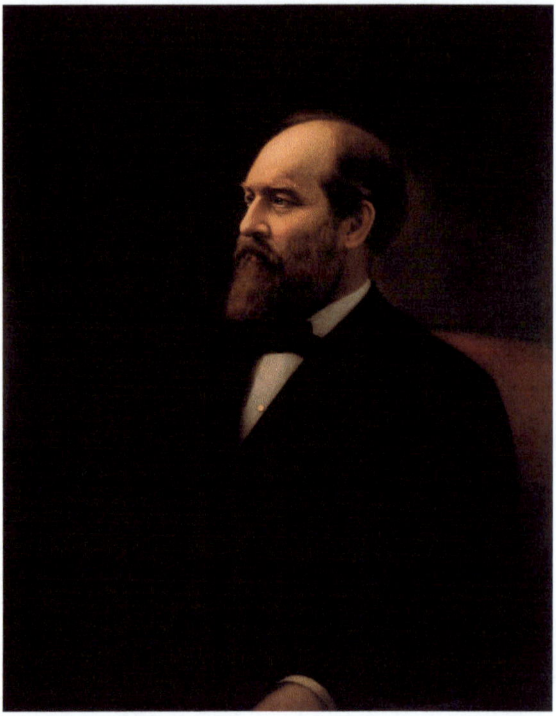

Fig. 4.1 James A. Garfield (public domain). *Source* Calvin curtis—http://www.whitehouseresearch.org/assetbank-whha/action/viewHome Official Presidential portrait of James Abram Garfield

Kentucky, which had recently been occupied by the Confederate Army. Despite being outnumbered, lacking artillery, and facing a renowned general with formal military training, Garfield and his men immediately set out to accomplish the task, which was decided a few months later at the Battle of Middle Creek. Thanks to Garfield's brilliant and daring strategy, the 42nd Regiment emerged victorious, permanently expelling the Confederates from Kentucky. This success earned him a promotion to General and made him a war hero. Ten months later he was re-elected to Congress and, at the request of Abraham Lincoln himself, left the army to devote himself to politics (Millard, 2011).

Despite concerns about abandoning his men on the battlefield, Garfield quickly realized that it was in Congress where his actions could have more significant and lasting effects. Thus, he devoted himself to promoting various initiatives that would earn him fame and recognition among his colleagues, including the resolution that allowed the *Free Movement of Blacks* throughout Washington DC and others aimed at funding the exploration and expansion of the country westward. Despite all his successes and growing reputation in Congress, Garfield, surprisingly, never sought to hold higher office within American politics. For 17 years, he limited himself to serving as a representative from northeastern Ohio, without ever attempting to test his strength or opportunities in more prominent positions (Peskin, 1978).

By 1880, Garfield was a widely recognized figure in American politics, primarily for three reasons: his solid values in a deeply corrupt environment, his apparent lack of personal ambition, and his exceptional oratory skills. The latter quality led John Sherman, Secretary of the Treasury and former Senator from Ohio, to ask Garfield to nominate him as the Republican Party's presidential candidate at the convention to be held in Chicago in June. (Millard, 2011) By June 1880, the Republican Party was deeply divided into two factions with sharply opposing views on how to conduct politics moving forward. On one side, the Stalwarts fervently defended the patronage system that had prevailed thus far, in which public offices and even state contracts were awarded at the discretion of party members and allies, based on their contributions to electoral victories and their relationships with those in power. On the other side, the Half-Breeds were reformers who opposed this system, believing it would ultimately lead to the downfall of the Republic, and advocated for a merit-based system. Sherman and Garfield belonged to this latter group. Amid this climate, the Chicago convention was set to determine the party's candidate for President of the United States (Millard C, 2011). In an event marked by shouting, jeers, insults, threats and attempted bribery, and in an atmosphere of total polarization, Garfield's speech in support of Sherman was the only moment of calm, reflection, and call for reason in pursuit of a greater good. The subsequent voting reflected the turmoil of the convention; after three days and more than forty ballots, there was still no consensus on a candidate. On the morning of the fourth day, without ever having been nominated, Garfield's name began to appear on the ballots. Despite his own opposition, as the day progressed, his candidacy gained momentum. In the afternoon, Sherman himself withdrew from the race to support him. By the end of the fourth day, James A. Garfield was unanimously chosen as the Republican Party's candidate for President of the United States. The ensuing campaign reflected this same spirit, as Garfield refused to participate in any political rallies, leaving the campaign in the hands of the Party and limiting himself to receiving anyone who wished to speak with him at his Ohio farm. His unconventional methods only increased his popularity in the eyes of the American public. The November election proved to be a mere formality, with the outcome already well known. (Millard, 2011).

The first months of Garfield's administration were marked by strong opposition from factions within his own party. True to his convictions, he decided to pursue an agenda focused on a series of laws and reforms aimed at ending the practice of patronage. Undeterred by criticism, rejection, and divisions within the Republican Party, Garfield continued to push forward, convinced that these measures were necessary for the country (Peskin, 1978).

On the morning of July 2, 1881, Garfield, accompanied by several members of his cabinet, headed to the Baltimore and Potomac railroad station in Washington, D.C., intending to take a train to New England, where he planned to enjoy a few days of vacation. At that time, there were no security measures in place for presidents, who traveled with a lack of protection unimaginable today. While waiting in the lounge, he was approached from behind by Charles Guiteau, who fired two shots at the president. The first bullet merely grazed Garfield's shoulder. The second entered through the lumbar region and lodged in the president's body. Amid screams of panic and the frantic flight of most of those present, Garfield collapsed to the ground. Guiteau was apprehended by one of the police officers at the station, while shouting, "I am a Stalwart of the Stalwarts." The assassin, a frustrated lawyer and preacher with a history of emotional instability and a member of the most radical faction of the Republicans, had supported Garfield's candidacy and, in line with the thesis he espoused, expected a reward for his assistance, specifically the consulship in Paris or Vienna. When his wishes were not granted, he decided that he had to eliminate Garfield to "save" the Republican Party and the nation (Millard, 2011).

Beyond the initial shock, Garfield's wounds were not fatal. After the initial assessment at the train station, the president was transported back to the White House, where, according to the prevailing medical knowledge of the time, all efforts were focused on extracting the bullet. In the following days, several physicians probed Garfield's wound with a multitude of instruments in numerous unsuccessful attempts to remove it. Even Alexander Graham Bell, who had recently introduced the telephone to the world, developed a device using magnets that also failed to achieve the desired result. The real problem, however, was something none of the attending physicians anticipated. All the examinations had been performed without asepsis (most without even gloves), using unsterilized instruments and unwashed hands. By the 1880s, Koch's postulates did not yet exist, and Pasteur's germ theory and Lister's work on the benefits of asepsis and antisepsis had only recently been published in Europe, where they were not yet universally accepted. In the United States, these ideas had become known only three years earlier, and most of the medical community neither believed in nor accepted their benefits. Garfield's wound became infected, resulting in abdominal sepsis. After 79 days of agony, on September 19, 1881, the president died. The autopsy concluded that Garfield died as a result of a severe intra-abdominal infection that led to rupture of the splenic artery. The bullet had not touched or damaged any vital structure (Bliss et al., 1881).

Garfield's death brought about enormous changes in the politics and social organization of the United States. Moreover, understanding the true cause of his death provided important lessons that persist to this day. On one hand, it helped to establish the principles of asepsis and antisepsis. On the other, it sparked a debate over what constitutes medical negligence. Even before Koch's postulates became universally known, Guiteau's defense would use this as an argument, claiming that he had "only shot the president, but it was the doctors who actually killed him" (Millard, 2011). Beyond this somewhat humorous defense attempt (Guiteau was convicted and hanged), the debate had only just begun. With the verification and acceptance of Lister's principles of asepsis and antisepsis, the discovery, visualization, and characterization of bacteria, a better understanding of Pasteur's germ theory, the development of sterilization methods, and the discovery and refinement of antibiotics, the errors made by the physicians who treated the president became increasingly evident and inexcusable. Today, this story is cited in books (Millard, 2011) and medical journals (Nguyen & Hufford, 2020; Paulson, 2006; Weiner, 2003) as a clear example of medical negligence. Virtually no text addressing the subject fails to reference Garfield's death.

It seems unfair to judge the physicians who treated him, as they acted according to the knowledge available at the time. Although Lister had already published his initial findings, all the knowledge underlying the assessment of these physicians emerged after Garfield's death. In fact, the incident itself led to broader and more rapid acceptance of asepsis and antisepsis. At the same time... would we think the same if, in the end, it had turned out that bacteria did not exist and that Lister was mistaken? Certainly not. So... why so much criticism? How can we so fervently blame physicians who acted in accordance with the knowledge available at the time? The answer likely lies in hindsight bias.

Definition

Hindsight bias is a cognitive error in which the likelihood of an event, situation, or outcome is judged after it has already occurred. Thus, once an event has taken place, it is believed to have been logical, expected, or easily predictable. Essentially, when looking back, facts and outcomes appear much more obvious and predictable than they actually were before they happened, regardless of the information available or what was thought about them prior to their occurrence.

Based on all current knowledge about bacteria, infections, asepsis and antisepsis, sterilization, and antibiotics, it is undeniable that the medical care received by President Garfield was inadequate. The mere thought of exploring a wound anywhere on the body without gloves, without prior cleaning, and with non-sterile instruments is an aberration. However, in 1880, almost all of this knowledge did not exist. The physicians responsible for the so-called "negligence" acted according to the knowledge and standards of their time. The outcomes were predictable, but only once the results were known and the knowledge explaining them had been developed. Judging actions and outcomes based on what happened and with information obtained later is a clear example of hindsight bias.

History

Hindsight bias was described by Fischhoff in 1975 (Fischhoff, 1975). In his research, he conducted a series of variations on a central experiment. In this experiment, participants were randomly divided into five groups, each of which was given a set of little-known real historical events or hypothetical medical scenarios to read, each with four possible outcomes that were, by design, mutually exclusive. For one of the groups, the reading ended at this point. The other four groups received an additional sentence, in which, without further explanation, they were told what had apparently occurred, corresponding to one of the four possible outcomes, with a different outcome for each group. Finally, participants were asked to estimate how likely, in their opinion, each of the outcomes was, regardless of whether they had been told the actual result. They were also required to list which aspects of the narrative had influenced, to a greater or lesser extent, their probability assignments. The results were unequivocal. Almost systematically, when an outcome was disclosed, it was considered at least twice as likely compared to the control group (which was not informed of any outcome). Moreover, the same aspects of the story were given more or less importance depending on the outcome revealed. Even more concerning, participants were unable to recognize the effect that the disclosed outcome had on their assessments and, therefore, believed that everyone should reach conclusions similar to their own.

Several subsequent studies replicated Fischhoff's initial results in different contexts and fields of knowledge. Among these, the work of Roese and Vohs stands out, as it provides insight into the underlying cognitive mechanisms responsible for the bias (Roese & Vohs, 2012).

Impact

Life involves a constant evaluation and reconsideration of the outcomes of actions, both individually and collectively. By directly impacting this ability, the effects of hindsight bias are manifold, extending across all facets of human activity. Among the most significant are:

At the Personal Level

1. **Overconfidence:** Believing that one could predict what happened leads to an excessive reliance on one's ability to foresee the future. This results in underestimating future risks and making decisions that are riskier than necessary, without adequately considering all possible options.
2. **Difficulty learning from mistakes:** If negative outcomes are inevitable, the motivation to analyze the causes of failure disappears, which limits the necessary process for improvement and adaptation.
3. **Biased evaluation of past decisions:** When outcomes are viewed as obvious in hindsight, it also impairs our ability to fairly assess our own decisions and those of others, leading to unjust judgments about ability and competence or to the inappropriate assignment of blame.
4. **Lack of understanding of complexity:** Rarely does a single action or decision lead to a specific outcome, especially when it comes to matters that are truly significant for the future. However, by simplifying past events and their outcomes as logical and/or inevitable, we lose the ability to assess the difficulty of situations and the multitude of variables that influence results, and we tend to seek simple solutions to complex problems.
5. **Memory distortion:** Retrospective bias leads to rewriting memories so that they fit the known outcome. As a result, opinions and predictions are remembered as being much more accurate and appropriate than they actually were.

At the Collective Level

1. **Misperception of public figures:** When the outcomes of any action are regarded as obvious or predictable, there is a tendency to judge leaders solely based on the results achieved, regardless of the complexity and uncertainty present at the time the decision was made or the role that chance may have played in the observed outcome.
2. **Loss of empathy:** When it is believed that the victims of a tragedy or those who have suffered a setback "should have known" or "could have taken precautions," collective empathy is diminished, fostering a culture in which victims ultimately become blamed for unfortunate outcomes.
3. **Inadequate Evaluation of History:** If researchers or historians are unable to put themselves in the shoes of the historical figures they are narrating, failing to grasp the complexity of the situations they faced and the knowledge available to them at the time decisions were made, any lesson drawn from the outcome will be inadequate and incorrect, ultimately distorting the value of historical figures by idealizing or demonizing them solely based on their achievements.

Examples in Medical and Surgical Practice

Medicine and surgery involve the constant evaluation of outcomes, as well as continuous learning based on these results. By affecting this capacity, hindsight bias exerts numerous effects on these disciplines. Among the most significant are:

1. Incorrect assessment of the success or failure of a given diagnosis or treatment strategy: When a particular positive or negative outcome is perceived as more obvious or predictable than it actually was, the evaluation process becomes completely distorted. Despite any uncertainty that may have existed, positive results make the diagnosis or treatment appear to have been "*clearly the best option from the start,*" while negative outcomes seem to have "*obviously been doomed to fail.*" This leads to an overestimation of the effectiveness of certain treatments and the undervaluation or dismissal of others.
2. Inadequate selection of future treatments: Successful outcomes lead to continued use of the same approach, based on the belief that "*if it worked once, it will work again,*" while negative results prompt avoidance due to the perception that "*they might fail.*" This simplistic view overlooks the necessary consideration of the various factors influencing the choice of a particular treatment, disregarding the specific characteristics that make a patient a better or worse candidate for these interventions.
3. Risk aversion and protocol overuse: In the face of poor outcomes, challenging cases, or limited treatment options, surgeons may become excessively cautious to avoid making seemingly "*obvious*" mistakes, opting for "*safer*" choices. This compromises clinical flexibility, as depending on the situation, some patients might benefit from more innovative and risk-taking strategies.

4. Biased perception of ability and expertise: When reviewing past cases, especially those with unfavorable outcomes, there is a tendency to fall into the "*I knew this was going to happen*" trap. This can lead to overconfidence if the outcome was positive ("*my intuition is excellent*") or to excessive and unfair self-criticism if it was negative ("*I should have seen the obvious*"). Both extremes distort the assessment of knowledge and abilities.
5. Inadequate evaluation of colleagues' or trainees' performance: If the outcome of a particular decision is known, it influences the way the process leading to that decision is analyzed. Judgments tend to be more lenient and the decision may be accepted as correct when the outcome is successful. For example, the analysis of a complication (such as postoperative bleeding) highlights the fact that the surgeon was "careless" with hemostatic measures.

How to Avoid Falling into Bias

1. **Consider and explain alternative outcomes:** Before assuming a result is obvious and inevitable, systematically consider other parallel scenarios and reason through the various factors that could have led to them. This mental exercise will make the actual outcome appear less predictable and more consistent with the uncertainty of the moment.
2. **Focus only on the information available at the time of the decision:** Regardless of the outcome, concentrate solely on the information that was available before the result occurred. Learn to disregard any information obtained afterward, especially that which is directly related to the outcome.
3. **Record predictions and expectations:** Before making any important decision, create a list of the information, beliefs, and arguments that lead to it, as well as the likely outcomes you expect, ranking them from most to least probable. Once the outcome is known, compare it and any new information obtained with the initial predictions. This will provide context for the analysis and allow you to assess whether something was truly "*known*" or "*obvious.*"
4. **Seek other perspectives:** Actively solicit the opinions of others, especially those with different viewpoints. Consult experts who are not directly involved in the situation. Encourage discussions within work groups.
5. **Taking responsibility for failures:** Hindsight bias can serve as a way to justify mistakes by believing that the negative outcome was inevitable regardless of our decisions, thus projecting a positive image of ourselves. In this regard, it is important to understand and accept that no one but oneself is responsible for both successes and mistakes.

References

Bliss, D. W., Barnes, J. K., & Woodward, J. J. (1881). Official record of the post-mortem examination of the body of president James a. *Garfield*. Henry C. Lea.
Fischhoff, B. (1975). Hindsight is not equal to foresight: The effect of outcome knowledge on judgment under uncertainty. *Journal of Experimental Psychology: Human Perception and Performance, 1*(3), 288–299. https://doi.org/10.1037/0096-1523.1.3.288
Millard, C. (2011). *Destiny of the republic: A tale of madness*. Knopf Doubleday Publishing Group. https://books.google.com.co/books?id=bRFQ74gYIPAC
Nguyen, C., & Hufford, T. (2020). Presidential assassinations: Historical review with current technology. *The American Surgeon, 86*(1), 2–7. https://www.ncbi.nlm.nih.gov/pubmed/32077409
Paulson, G. (2006). Death of a president and his assassin—Errors in their diagnosis and autopsies. *Journal of the History of the Neurosciences, 15*(2), 77–91. https://doi.org/10.1080/096470490953455
Peskin, A. (1978). *Garfield: A biography*. Kent State University Press.
Roese, N. J., & Vohs, K. D. (2012). Hindsight bias. *Perspectives on Psychological Science, 7*(5), 411–426. https://doi.org/10.1177/1745691612454303
Weiner, B. K. (2003). The case of James a. Garfield: A historical perspective. *Spine (Phila Pa 1976), 28*(10), E183–E186. https://doi.org/10.1097/01.BRS.0000062002.52586.04

Chapter 5
Attention Bias. Prefrontal Lobotomy and Mental Illness

The Problem

In May 1937, Egas Moniz (Tan & Yip, 2014) (Fig. 5.1), a renowned professor of neurology at the University of Lisbon known for his contributions to cerebral angiography, two-time Nobel Prize in Medicine nominee, and veteran politician, published an article presenting his results with a new procedure called **prefrontal leucotomy** for the treatment of mental illness. (Moniz, 1994) Together with neurosurgeon Almeida Lima, he performed the first leucotomy on March 3, 1936, after observing the results of an experiment conducted by John Fulton and Carlyle Jacobsen at Yale University, which demonstrated behavioral changes in primates following removal of the frontal lobes. In a monograph, he shared his initial findings in 18 patients before the Paris Neurological Society.

The procedure consisted of two lateral trepanations followed by the incision of the prefrontal white matter, aiming to disconnect this area from the rest of the brain. With successful outcomes in only three out of eighteen schizophrenic patients, Moniz concluded that "the *facts speak for themselves*," recommending the operation as a simple and safe solution, thus giving rise to a new branch of surgery and psychiatry: psychosurgery. Although he noted that some "*deteriorated patients obtain slight or no benefit from the treatment*," his focus was specifically on those who showed improvement.

Across the Atlantic, in the United States, Walter J. Freeman II (Caruso & Sheehan, 2017) (Fig. 5.2), then head of the Department of Neurology at George Washington University, and James Watts, a young neurosurgeon, performed the first leucotomy on September 4, 1936, becoming devoted advocates of this new treatment. Within six years, they had already performed more than 200 procedures. Freeman and Watts introduced the first modification to the surgical technique, which became known as the prefrontal lobotomy, a major surgical procedure performed under general anesthesia. Later, Freeman further modified it into an office-based procedure, accessing the frontal lobe through a hole in the roof of the orbit (transorbital lobotomy).

A. Sanabria and C. Betancourt, *Cognitive Biases in Surgical Practice*,
https://doi.org/10.1007/978-3-032-20377-9_5

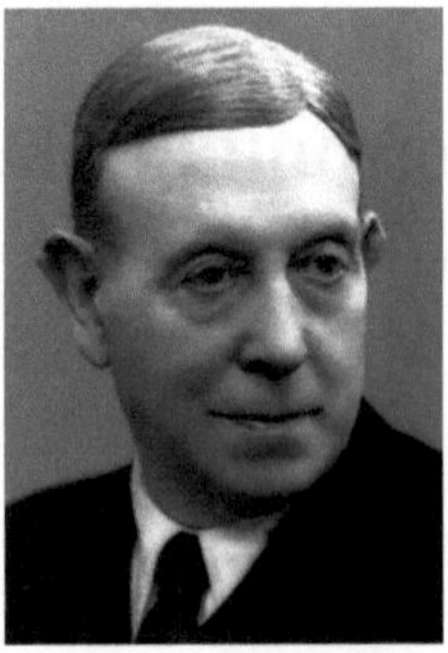

Fig. 5.1 António Caetano de Moniz (public domain). Unknown—Artico M, Spoletini M, Fumagalli L, Biagioni F, Ryskalin L, Fornai F, Salvati M, Frati A, Pastore FS and Taurone S (2017) Egas Moniz: 90 Years (1927–2017) since Cerebral Angiography. Front. Neuroanat. 11:81. https://doi.org/10.3389/fnana.2017.00081

According to Freeman, the initial results showed a 63% effectiveness in controlling mental symptoms, less than 1% complication rate, and only 3% mortality. (Freeman, 1950) Thanks to Freeman's conviction, charisma, and the significant support of the press, this surgery was promoted as miraculous. In 1942, Freeman and Watts published their textbook *Psychosurgery*, which provided theoretical foundation to justify lobotomy. Metaphors such as "*transforming wild animals into gentle creatures*" were coined by the authors and communicated to the press to gain public support. Publicity thus became an incentive to perform the procedure, and anecdotal reports of spectacular cures motivated families and individuals to consider this option. Publications became milestones, such as the article published by H. Dannecker, a former patient, in the magazine *Coronet* entitled "*Psychosurgery Cured Me*." Soon, other renowned American physicians such as James Lyerly, Mesrop Tarumianz, and Harold Palmer adopted the technique and expanded its indications. The procedure was quickly implemented in England in 1940, in Sweden in 1944, and in France in 1946. (Ogren, 2013).

The indications gradually broadened to include, in addition, patients with schizophrenia, depression, anxiety, obsessive-compulsive disorder, bipolar disorder, intractable pain, epilepsy, asthma, and even gastric ulcer disease.

Despite optimistic opinions, since 1941, the *American Medical Association* (AMA, 1941), in a panel discussion, highlighted the weaknesses in the information provided by the main proponents of lobotomy. Nevertheless, by 1950, more than 10,000 lobotomies had been performed in the United States, with a similar number in the United Kingdom.

In 1950, a growing number of critical voices raised concerns about the low effectiveness of the treatment. Despite early warnings from some physicians (Diefenbach et al., 1999) regarding the lack of solid data to justify this surgery, most of the scientific community saw only the advantages of the therapy in the absence of other effective treatments for mental illness. Furthermore, the alarming increase in the number of patients remaining in asylums and psychiatric hospitals, and confined in

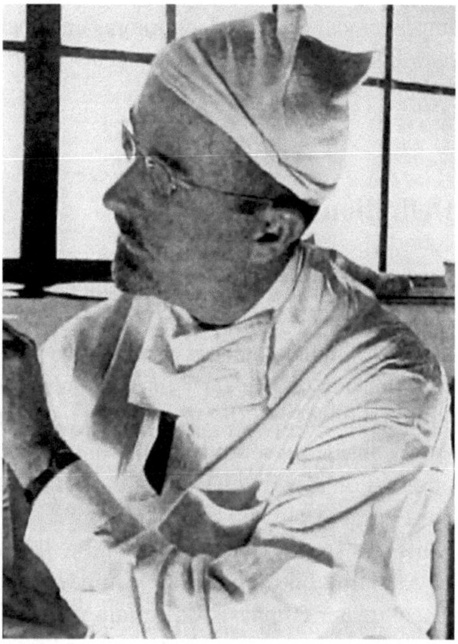

Fig. 5.2 Walter Freeman (public domain). Photograph by Harris A. Ewing—Saturday Evening Post, May 24, 1941, pages 18–19. https://commons.wikimedia.org/wiki/File:Walter_Jackson_Freeman_II.jpg

their own homes after treatment, especially after the end of the Second World War, accelerated the doubts in this type of therapy.

The wave of criticism, however, was partially calmed by the awarding of the Nobel Prize in Medicine to Egas Moniz in 1949 "*for his discovery of the therapeutic value of leucotomy in certain psychoses*." The introduction of chlorpromazine, the first antipsychotic drug, in 1954, dealt the final blow to lobotomy, although Freeman continued to defend it until his death.

The excessive focus on successful cases (Terrier et al., 2019), promoted by physicians such as Freeman and facilitated by newspapers and popular magazines that advertised the treatment as "*astonishing,*" "*spectacular*" or "*a new opportunity in life*"; as an alternative for treating criminal behavior, and even as a means of controlling individuals deemed undesirable or antisocial (Ogren, 2013), is a clear demonstration of **attention bias.** Captivated by the positive outcomes, these same media (Afkhami et al., 2022) rarely discussed the risks, complications, or adverse outcomes, and when they did, they used euphemistic or minimizing language or even implied them as desirable effects. In other instances, when weighing risks and benefits, the risks were underestimated or tolerated considering the alternative of a mentally unsatisfying life. Even high-profile cases of adverse outcomes, such as that of Rosemary Kennedy, sister of the President of the United States, were mentioned only very superficially.

Subsequently studying the phenomenon, Afkhami et al. (2022), in an analysis of the content of scientific articles related to lobotomy, demonstrated that there were more references to the positive aspects of the therapy, such as safety and precision, improvement of mental symptoms and social functioning,and effects on psychiatric care institutions, than to the negative aspects, such as complications and adverse effects.

Definition

Attention is defined as a state in which most cognitive resources (perception, memory, reasoning, processing, etc.) (Harvey, 2019) are focused on certain specific aspects of the environment and not on others.

Attention bias refers to the tendency to prioritize the processing of salient external stimuli (images, words, data, etc.) or internal stimuli (hunger, pain, emotion, etc.) over those considered neutral. In this context, decision-making is influenced by the degree of attention a particular stimulus can elicit in an individual. Thus, if a stimulus is more attractive, it will occupy a more significant role in the decision-making process, while less salient or neutral stimuli will have reduced or negligible relevance.

Attention bias significantly impacts decision-making by causing individuals to place greater emphasis on certain types of information while downplaying others, leading to a loss of perspective regarding the broader context in which the decision is made. In some contexts, this phenomenon has been referred to as *"tunnel vision."* (Mack & Rock, 1998).

The characteristics of everyday stimuli such as food (color, taste, smell), news (type of image, associated music), advertisements (models, setting), or messages on social media (font size, speed at which images change) focus attention on these aspects and lead to the neglect of other equally important features, such as the caloric content of food, the existence of alternative explanations for news, the disadvantages of an advertised product, or the intent of an agent to access personal information through social networks. In addition, certain personal traits can direct attention to particular stimuli, as seen in the increased attention to threatening stimuli among anxious individuals or to negative aspects among people with depression (Abado et al., 2020). Similarly, it has been shown that in internal states such as hunger, people pay greater attention to food-related stimuli, and that in certain addictions such as smoking, smokers exhibit a heightened response to tobacco-related cues.

In the case of prefrontal lobotomy, the conviction of Moniz and Freeman regarding the procedure's effectiveness as a cure for mental illness, where only the benefits were emphasized, along with the widespread involvement of the media, which reported exclusively on successful cases even in the face of well-founded criticism, can be explained by attention bias. We are already familiar with the disastrous consequences.

History

Psychologist John Ridley Stroop, from the Peabody College of Education and Human Development at Vanderbilt University, is recognized as the first to introduce an experimental method for measuring attention bias in 1935, giving rise to what is now known as the *Stroop effect*. (Stroop, 1935) This effect refers to the interference that occurs between reading the name of an object and the object itself, as demonstrated by assessing response speed using a table in which color names and the colors in which they were printed were swapped. This showed that focusing attention on one feature impairs the processing of other features.

In 1984, Ian Gotlib and Douglas McCann (Gotlib & McCann, 1984) expanded the original *Stroop* experiment to include the interpretation of emotionally charged words, demonstrating that individuals with depressive traits exhibited greater latency in naming the color of emotionally negative words. Finally, Collin MacLeod, Andrew Mathews, and Philip Tata (MacLeod et al., 1986) from the University of London described the *dot-probe task*, which assesses reaction speed to neutral or threatening stimuli, revealing faster responses to stimuli perceived as dangerous, indicating selective attention to such stimuli.

It is assumed that **attention bias** is an evolutionary response to the need to remain alert to certain stimuli that may threaten survival (such as animals or weapons) or enhance reproductive opportunities (such as beauty), at the expense of less dangerous stimuli. (Haselton et al., 2016) Due to improvements in living conditions and the progressive absence of potentially lethal stimuli, excessive and selective attention to non-threatening stimuli can lead to poor decision-making.

Impact

Modern life involves an abundance of stimuli, and individuals need to prioritize this information efficiently. Since attention is one of the most important factors in decision-making, focusing it on relevant aspects is key to making sound decisions. Conversely, if attention is directed toward irrelevant elements that are mistakenly assumed to be of greater benefit or risk, this can lead to catastrophic decision errors. Thus, the effects of bias are expected to be multiple and diverse. Among the most significant are:

At the Personal Level:

1. **Limited consideration of options:** Focusing the attention on certain options or stimuli, which hinders the rational analysis of the full range of possibilities.
2. **Disproportionate Influence of Internal and External States:** Several factors such as personality traits (anxiety, depression), mood states (stress, fear, sadness), past experiences, etc., can divert attention, thereby affecting the decisions made at a given moment.

3. **Distortion of reality based on interests and expectations:** Interest in specific topics, driven by personal factors (such as medical specialty), institutional factors (a hospital specialized in cancer care), social factors (easy access to certain technologies), or cultural factors (the importance placed on aesthetic outcomes in the postoperative period), along with the belief that these are highly significant in decision-making, can focus attention on certain aspects to the detriment of others.
4. **Excessive cognitive load:** When faced with decision-making situations involving many variables acting simultaneously, there is a tendency to select only a few of these variables to analyze the problem, usually those that require less cognitive effort, while neglecting others that are equally important.

At the Collective Level:

1. **Stereotype Formation:** By focusing attention solely on certain behaviors or attributes consistent with a particular model, while ignoring information that challenges it, contributes to the maintenance of prejudices, and affects social interactions.
2. **Creation of Opinion Bubbles:** When the media or opinion leaders (political, cultural, and social) decide which topics or news items to focus on, they influence what society considers important, urgent, or relevant, directing public attention toward certain issues and away from others that may be equally or even more significant.

Examples in Medical and Surgical Practice

In medicine and surgery, decisions are made every minute throughout the workday, and these can be influenced by attention bias. Among the most significant cases are:

1. Emotion-driven decisions that focus attention on secondary situations, such as when a dispute with a colleague occurs during a complication review meeting and attention is subsequently directed toward the points of contention rather than objectively assessing the facts.
2. Refusal to introduce new treatment alternatives due to an exclusive emphasis on risks without considering the benefits. For example, the initial rejection of laparoscopic cholecystectomy because of a 0.1% increase in bile duct injury rates, without considering the deaths prevented by avoiding surgical wound complications. (Büchler et al., 1995).
3. Excessive search for signs and symptoms using clinical and paraclinical methods to prevent recurrence of a previous complication. For instance, ordering multiple abdominal imaging studies (ultrasound, CT scan, etc.) after a complication resulting from a diagnostic error in a case of acute appendicitis. (Pei et al., 2018).
4. Use of technologies without scientific evidence of effectiveness but which are employed because the surgeon previously had patients with extraordinary outcomes, without considering those who did not benefit or are not candidates for

the same intervention. For example, a surgeon who, after successfully performing a laparoscopic gastrectomy, insists on always using this approach, overlooking cases that would benefit from open surgery.

5. Active search for new cases of a particular disease when the surgeon has just completed training in a specific skill or has recently attended a conference. For example, the relationship between the density of endocrine surgeons and the use of thyroid ultrasound for nodule detection. (McDow et al., 2022).

How to Avoid Falling into Bias?

Among the strategies that can help protect against the negative impact of attention bias are: (Webster et al., 2021)

1. **Maintain focus on the present moment:** Since some of the factors that contribute to attention bias stem from previously experienced situations, keeping attention on the present situation helps prevent the inadvertent influence that past experiences may exert on the focus of attention. Practicing brief moments of *mindfulness* before making a critical decision or during episodes of stress helps to refocus attention.
2. **Use tools for identifying variables and critical factors in decision-making:** One way to avoid the inadvertent effect that may arise from focusing excessively on a particular factor when deciding is the routine use of checklists, objective decision-making tools, and brainstorming. (Gawande, 2009).
3. **Identify one's own mental frameworks and how they operate:** Surgeons' preferences regarding risk (aversion or propensity) are not fixed and vary between situations. The same surgeon may behave in a risk-averse mode in a specific situation (choosing a new treatment) and be risk-seeking (opting for an invasive diagnostic method) in others. Belonging to one of these frameworks leads to focusing attention on particular characteristics of an alternative. Risk-averse individuals tend to focus their attention on risk probabilities, while risk-seeking individuals focus more on outcomes. The same occurs if attention is directed toward gains (the option with the greatest gains will be chosen) or toward losses (the option with the greatest losses will be rejected). (Hu et al., 2024).
4. **Engage individuals with different viewpoints and obtain second opinions:** Attention bias is ubiquitous, and even when its existence and effects are known, it is difficult to recognize when it is operating. When facing a decision, one alternative is to apply the "*devil's advocate*" strategy, involving a person and giving them the authority to criticize the proposed alternatives. Another approach is to form groups with individuals who have divergent or complementary perspectives, so they can evaluate the selected options.

References

Abado, E., Richter, T., & Okon-Singer, H. (2020). Chapter 2 - attention bias toward negative stimuli. In T. Aue & H. Okon-Singer (Eds.), *Cognitive biases in health and psychiatric disorders* (pp. 19–40). Academic Press. https://doi.org/10.1016/B978-0-12-816660-4.00002-7

Afkhami, A. A., Fatollahi, J. J., Peace, M. A., & Yadgar, R. J. (2022). Spinning lobotomy: A conventional content analysis of articles by the pioneers of the procedure in the United States. *SSM - Mental Health, 2*, 100123. https://doi.org/doi:10.1016/j.ssmmh.2022.100123

AMA. (1941). Neurosurgical treatment of certain abnormal mental states: Panel discussion at Cleveland session. *Journal of the American Medical Association, 117*(7), 517–527. https://doi.org/10.1001/jama.1941.72820330004007

Büchler, M.W., Frei, E., Klaiber, C., Krähenbühl, L. Five Years of Laparoscopic Cholecystectomy: A Reappraisal: International Meeting, Bern, May 1995. (1996). S.Karger AG. doi:https://doi.org/10.1159/isbn.978-3-318-04152-1.

Caruso, J. P., & Sheehan, J. P. (2017). Psychosurgery, ethics, and media: A history of Walter Freeman and the lobotomy. *Neurosurgical Focus, 43*(3), E6. https://doi.org/10.3171/2017.6.FOCUS17257

Diefenbach, G. J., Diefenbach, D., Baumeister, A., & West, M. (1999). Portrayal of lobotomy in the popular press: 1935-1960. *Journal of the History of the Neurosciences, 8*(1), 60–69. https://doi.org/10.1076/jhin.8.1.60.1766

Freeman, W. (1950). Psychosurgery. *Journal of the National Medical Association, 42*(4), 206–209. https://www.ncbi.nlm.nih.gov/pubmed/15428888

Gawande, A. (2009). *The checklist manifesto*. Metropolitan Books.

Gotlib, I. H., & McCann, C. D. (1984). Construct accessibility and depression: An examination of cognitive and affective factors. *Journal of Personality and Social Psychology, 47*(2), 427–439. https://doi.org/10.1037//0022-3514.47.2.427

Harvey, P. D. (2019). Domains of cognition and their assessment *dialogues clin Neurosci, 21* (3), 227-237. https://doi.org/10.31887/DCNS.2019.21.3/pharvey

Haselton, M. G., Nettle, D., & Murray, D. R. (2016). The evolution of cognitive bias. In The handbook of evolutionary psychology: Integrations, *Vol. 2, 2nd ed.* (pp. 968–987). John Wiley & Sons, Inc.

Hu, M., Chang, R., Sui, X., & Gao, M. (2024). Attention biases the process of risky decision-making: Evidence from eye-tracking. *Psych J, 13*(2), 157–165. https://doi.org/10.1002/pchj.724

Mack, A., & Rock, I. (1998). Inattentional Blindness. *The MIT Press*. https://doi.org/10.7551/mitpress/3707.001.0001

MacLeod, C., Mathews, A., & Tata, P. (1986). Attentional bias in emotional disorders. *Journal of Abnormal Psychology, 95*(1), 15–20. https://doi.org/10.1037//0021-843x.95.1.15

McDow, A. D., Lanzotti, N., Zahnd, W. E., MacKinney, E. C., Angelos, P., Mellinger, J. D., & Ganai, S. (2022). Impact of endocrinologist and surgeon density on well-differentiated thyroid cancer survival. *The American Surgeon, 88*(11), 2626–2632. https://doi.org/10.1177/00031348221091958

Moniz, E. (1994). Prefrontal leucotomy in the treatment of mental disorders. 1937. *The American Journal of Psychiatry, 151*(6 Suppl), 236–239. https://doi.org/10.1176/ajp.151.6.236

Ogren, K. (2013). Portrayals of lobotomy in American and Swedish media. *Progress in Brain Research, 206*, 201–217. https://doi.org/10.1016/B978-0-444-63364-4.00028-4

Pei, K. Y., Healy, J., & Davis, K. A. (2018). Surgeons overestimate postoperative complications and mortality compared to the National Surgical Quality Improvement Project risk calculator. *The Journal of Surgical Research, 225*, 95–100. https://doi.org/10.1016/j.jss.2018.01.008

Stroop, J. R. (1935). Studies of interference in serial verbal reactions. *Journal of Experimental Psychology, 18*(6), 643–662. https://doi.org/10.1037/h0054651

Tan, S. Y., & Yip, A. (2014). Antonio Egas Moniz (1874-1955): Lobotomy pioneer and Nobel laureate. *Singapore Medical Journal, 55*(4), 175–176. https://doi.org/10.11622/smedj.2014048

Terrier, L. M., Leveque, M., & Amelot, A. (2019). Brain lobotomy: A historical and moral dilemma with no alternative? *World Neurosurgery, 132*, 211–218. https://doi.org/10.1016/j.wneu.2019.08.254
Webster, C. S., Taylor, S., & Weller, J. M. (2021). Cognitive biases in diagnosis and decision making during anesthesia and intensive care. *BJA Educ, 21*(11), 420–425. https://doi.org/10.1016/j.bjae.2021.07.004

Chapter 6
Availability Bias. The Angelina Jolie Effect

The Problem

In the first half of 2013, actress and model Angelina Jolie shocked the globe. In an opinion essay headlined "*My Medical Decision*," the actress, considered one of the most beautiful in the world, explained the process she went through while deciding to undergo a prophylactic or risk-reducing bilateral mastectomy. The reason? Concerned about her mother's premature death at the age of 56 because of breast cancer, she had a genetic test and tested positive for the BRCA1 gene mutation. Her physicians advised her that this mutation, together with her family history, put her at an 87% risk of having breast cancer. She elected to have the operation, and her risk was reduced to less than 1%. In the article, she described in detail the three operations (mastectomy and reconstructions) that she had undergone, adding that in the end, she was still the same, with just "*a few small scars*." At the same time, she asserted that her femininity had not changed at all. Finally, she advised any woman with a history of breast or ovarian cancer to seek information and medical care, not to live in "*the shadow of cancer*," and to be aware that there were possibilities for "*timely*" detection and treatment (Jolie, 2013).

Her piece had an instant effect. The willingness of a well-known female professional to endure a mutilating procedure suggested that the genetic abnormality and its repercussions were significant. In what has become known as "*the Angelina Jolie effect*," online searches for genetic mutations in breast cancer and its treatment increased dramatically. In the first 15 days following publication, the number of genetic tests for the BRCA mutation in the United States jumped by 64% (Johnson, 2016). In the second half of 2013, the number of genetic tests done on American women climbed from 0.7 to 1.13 per 100,000 women, a trend that was sustained for the next three years (Desai & Jena, 2016). Furthermore, the number of women diagnosed with early-stage breast cancer who chose bilateral total mastectomy over more conservative and equally effective treatment choices increased significantly,

A. Sanabria and C. Betancourt, *Cognitive Biases in Surgical Practice*,
https://doi.org/10.1007/978-3-032-20377-9_6

regardless of whether the patient carried the mutation. Many of the less aggressive and equally acceptable treatment alternatives for breast cancer were rejected at the request of patients. On a more personal level, several women hosted parties after being diagnosed with the mutation and booked for bilateral mastectomy as a celebration of the cancer-free life they would now be able to lead (Mapes, 2014).

However, once the initial euphoria had dissipated, data began to come up that put the new conduct into doubt. On the one hand, the BCRA mutation was not new in the medical community. Discovered in 1994, serious research revealed that its frequency in the general population was about 0.2% to 0.3%, accounting for less than 10% of all breast cancers (Nelson et al., 2014). Furthermore, while the overall number of bilateral mastectomies rose, the proportion of mastectomies done in women who underwent genetic testing did not rise considerably, confirming the mutation's rarity (Liede et al., 2018). Similarly, there were other treatment choices for women with the mutation, such as active surveillance, which eliminated the need for mastectomy. Finally, the genetic test was not inexpensive (USD $3000 in 2013), and the rise in costs for the health system was expected to be $14 million in the second half of 2013 (Johnson, 2016).

A few years later, the medical community realized that the concern caused by Jolie's writing had resulted in an unjustified rise in genetic testing, a disproportionate increase in total mastectomies, and the abandonment of alternative, equally effective therapeutic choices. At the same time, there was growing concern about the impact of the false sense of security on women who did not carry the mutation (the vast majority of those who chose genetic testing), who now considered themselves immune to breast cancer and did not undergo established screening and early detection tests. Later, stories emerged of women who chose a bilateral mastectomy due to equivocal genetic test findings, while already knowing they had no chance of getting cancer (Moyer, 2014). As a result, the scientific community recognized the importance of intervening in the media's content to educate women and calm collective excitement. In the fourth quarter of 2015, several papers were published in the world's largest newspapers reporting on the existence of the BRCA mutation, its association with breast cancer, and whether a preventative mastectomy is necessary. Finally, on October 24, 2019, Jolie published a fresh piece in Time magazine in which she reviewed her choice considering recent scientific knowledge and said unequivocally that there were alternative treatment options besides hers and that each case had to be individualized (Jolie, 2019).

When reading this story, it's tough not to wonder how this occurred. The BRCA mutation's presence and prevalence, as well as its link to breast cancer, were previously well understood. Treatments for people in the early stages of breast cancer were well known. Total mastectomy was becoming less popular in favor of less mutilating procedures like quadrantectomy. Breast cancer therapy was perhaps the clearest illustration in oncology of how multimodality may be built around a disease, resulting in good outcomes, an outstanding long-term prognosis, and minimal functional and cosmetic consequences. How might an individual's experience in a highly uncommon setting cause so much commotion? Could it be that all it takes is a well-known name in a widely distributed media to readily modify long-standing medical practices? The solution to these issues is found in one of the most explored cognitive biases: the availability bias.

Definition

This cognitive bias is defined as the process by which the brain assesses the frequency and/or significance of an event or occurrence based on how easily it comes to memory. As with other cognitive biases, a tough decision is substituted by an easier one: the difficult one is looking for facts to assess how common or significant a situation or incident is, and the easier one is how simple it is to recall such a scenario or event. Thus, dramatic occurrences (accidents, natural catastrophes), striking events (involving renowned individuals such as politicians, sports, movie stars, and so on), extensively publicized media events (pictures, videos), or personal or family experiences are perceived as more common and important than they are. On the other hand, ordinary occurrences that receive little attention because they are so regular are neglected or dismissed as irrelevant. This bias explained "*the Angelina Jolie effect*" in the given story. A rare incident with a high chance of mortality is mixed with the viewpoint of a celebrity who sees an inflated danger of death, resulting in it being perceived as much more common and important than it is, with all the repercussions and impact previously mentioned.

History

This bias was first described by Tversky and Kahneman in 1973 (Tversky & Kahneman, 1973). In the paper, the authors provided the findings of ten psychological studies conducted in various circumstances that conclusively demonstrated its existence. Several subsequent articles have validated similar conclusions. Paul Slovic's studies stand out, as he established in an experiment in which participants voted on the most prevalent causes of death between two distinct options, that when calculating the risk, the same inaccuracy occurs (*The perception of risk*, 2000). Norbert Schwarz's work concluded that availability affected estimates through two mechanisms: the number of events that could be remembered (the greater the number, the greater the probability and/or risk), and the ease with which these events were remembered (the easier, the greater the probability and/or risk) (Schwarz et al., 1991).

Impact

Availability bias influences how you perceive and think about the world around you in several ways. Among the most significant are:

Personally

1. **Estimates of an event's likelihood (frequency):** Situations that are memorable because they are dramatic, startling, extensively broadcast by the media, personal, and so on are thought to be far more common than they are. In turn, typical occurrences that lack the aforementioned traits are considered unusual. The prevalent notion is that an aviation accident is more likely to result in death than a car collision, although the former occurs far less frequently.
2. **Risk estimates:** Events that are easily recalled and have the potential to cause losses are considered more frequent and significant than those that do not. Following an earthquake or other natural disaster, sales of insurance that covers damages from catastrophic occurrences increase, only to nearly evaporate months later.
3. **The importance of information sources (news in the media):** If the brain is innately susceptible to dramatic and spectacular circumstances, which influences how we see the world, we should pay more attention to what we see, hear, and read. The news on television and radio, newspapers, and social networks are usually full of tragic, overwhelming, shocking, and suggestive situations or events involving well-known and/or important people, which are usually accompanied by explicit videos and vivid audio. Despite being extremely rare events, they are easily recorded in memories. However, when you reflect on these events later, the availability bias causes them to be perceived as much more common and significant than they are, distorting the true appraisal of the situation. Given this knowledge, it is crucial to ask: To what degree is it worthwhile to use these sources of information? Are we employing them correctly, or do they influence us?

On a Collective Level

1. **Availability cascades**: According to Timur Kuran and Cass Sunstein, (Kuran & Sunstein, 1998) an availability cascade is a self-sustaining chain of events that begins with a small number of individuals persuading the media to publicize a modest or even insignificant event or situation, eventually leading to fear and mass hysteria. This encourages large-scale social and/or governmental initiatives. Thus, a minor condition that only affects a small number of people escalates into a problem for a region, a country, or even the entire planet, resulting in large-scale activities that affect the lives of most people. The "**Angelina Jolie effect**" is an obvious illustration of this phenomenon.

Examples from Medical and Surgical Practice

Availability bias exists in all facets of the surgeon's professional activity. The effects of availability operate in all areas of surgical practice; nevertheless, they are not usually recognized for what they are, even though they have direct repercussions for both the doctor and the patient. These may be mentioned:

At Diagnosis

1. Early identification of certain indolent illnesses when detection is overemphasized, as in some awareness campaigns. Consider the recent increase in the incidence of thyroid cancer.
2. Excessive screening for common illnesses, such as when laboratory-based preventative check-ups are encouraged. Consider the indiscriminate use of prostate-specific antigen (PSA) in asymptomatic males.
3. Indiscriminate use of diagnostic tests in instances when the benefit is little, yet they are heavily marketed. For example, use genetic tests (personal genomics) to reveal discoveries of unmodifiable and low-impact mutations.

During the Treatment

1. Excessive usage of innovative technology, heavily promoted by the industry, with no major advantages for patients. For example, nerve monitors are used indiscriminately during parotid and thyroid procedures.
2. The prescription of more expensive pharmaceuticals with no benefits or just slight advantages over cheaper alternatives, but which have been frequently promoted at dinners or holiday events. For example, a medicine may be prescribed following a visit by a representative of the pharmaceutical business that supplies it.
3. The use of innovative treatment systems, but without clear proof that supports their benefits, which has been made recently available for demonstration. For example, Indication of a novel robotic operation following participation in a videoconference about its effective usage in a medical center on the opposite side of the globe.

When Establishing the Prognosis

1. The use of disease-specific tests or indicators following an event with more prominent speakers. For example: The count of circulating malignant cells in serum following treatment.
2. The obligation to obtain more imaging exams following the publication of a journalistic narrative in which an illness was "miraculously" discovered and saved a person's life. For example: The use of PET-CT as a tool "to detect all cancers".
3. The application of event probability to a case recently addressed at a decision board or morbidity and mortality meeting. For example, after discovering one uncommon or occasional occurrence, it is common to believe that they frequently occur in pairs or clusters.

How can you Prevent Falling into this Bias?

1. **Always doubt your first gut:** This advice will be repeated throughout this book. The first step in avoiding bias is to constantly doubt the initial thought that our brain presents to us. Although this is not always the case, and intuitions are sometimes true, it is most probable that when evaluating the frequency of an occurrence or the likelihood of a risk, the first thought that comes to mind is a product of availability.
2. **Determine the base rates:** The base rate is the chance of an event or scenario occurring in the absence of any other conditioning element. In today's globalized society, these probabilities have been estimated for nearly every known event and are available to everybody. As a result, if any phenomenon must be addressed, regardless of our intuition or the security we may have in it, we should always reference the base rate and begin any investigation there.
3. **In-depth study and knowledge of the illness and/or scenario:** As previously said, the greatest strategy to minimize bias is to be as familiar with the condition or occurrence as possible. As a result, time should always be set aside to thoroughly research and comprehend the illness, therapy, or procedure under consideration.
4. **Use information sources correctly:** As previously stated, the media and social networks provide information that favors availability bias. Therefore, correct usage is crucial. In this regard, anytime a disease, therapy, or other topic is examined or evaluated, serious, solid sources with statistical rigor should be considered (meta-analysis, systematic reviews, recommendations for management from major scientific bodies, etc.). Similarly, look for and acquire tools that enable critical analysis of literature.
5. **Use availability to your advantage:** According to Norbert Schwarz's research, the availability bias is made up of two components: the number of events we can recall and the ease with which we remember them. If recalling events becomes more difficult than expected, we will gradually abandon our initial assumption. In this manner, after the initial intuition comes, note the occasions when you can remember that the circumstance or incident occurred. If intuition is true, recalling multiple occurrences will be quite easy. Otherwise, the brain will rapidly realize it has fooled itself and modify its view.

References

Desai, S., & Jena, A. B. (2016). Do celebrity endorsements matter? Observational study of BRCA gene testing and mastectomy rates after Angelina Jolie's New York times editorial. *BMJ, 355*, i6357. https://doi.org/10.1136/bmj.i6357

Johnson, C. (2016, December 15). The unintended consequence of Angelina Jolie's viral breast cancer essay. *The Washington Post*, 1. https://www.washingtonpost.com/news/wonk/wp/2016/12/15/why-doctors-cant-ignore-celebrities-the-angelina-jolie-effect/

Jolie, A. (2013, May 14). My medical choice. *The New York Times*, 1. https://www.nytimes.com/2013/05/15/opinion/angelina-jolies-preventive-surgery.html

Jolie, A. (2019, October 24). Angelina Jolie: Medical advances in women's health are important. But they're only part of the picture. *Time*. https://time.com/5709290/angelina-jolie-cancer-research-prevention/

Kuran, T., & Sunstein, C. R. (1998). Availability cascades and risk regulation. *Stanford Law Review, 51*, 683.

Liede, A., Cai, M., Crouter, T. F., Niepel, D., Callaghan, F., & Evans, D. G. (2018). Risk-reducing mastectomy rates in the US: A closer examination of the Angelina Jolie effect. *Breast Cancer Research and Treatment, 171*(2), 435–442. https://doi.org/10.1007/s10549-018-4824-9

Mapes, D. (2014). The Angelina Jolie effect: One year later. *Fred Hutchinson Cancer Center*. Retrieved October 7, 2025, from https://www.fredhutch.org/en/news/center-news/2014/05/the-angelina-jolie-effect%2D%2Done-year-later.html

Moyer, J. (2014, September 13). Dueling studies: The 'Angelina Jolie effect' is influencing women fighting cancer. *The Washington Post*, 1. https://www.washingtonpost.com/news/morning-mix/wp/2014/09/03/study-the-angelina-effect-is-helping-women-beat-breast-cancer/

Nelson, H. D., Pappas, M., Zakher, B., Mitchell, J. P., Okinaka-Hu, L., & Fu, R. (2014). Risk assessment, genetic counseling, and genetic testing for BRCA-related cancer in women: A systematic review to update the U.S. preventive services task force recommendation. *Annals of Internal Medicine, 160*(4), 255–266. https://doi.org/10.7326/M13-1684

Schwarz, N., Bless, H., Strack, F., Klumpp, G., Rittenauer-Schatka, H., & Simons, A. (1991). Ease of retrieval as information: Another look at the availability heuristic. *Journal of Personality and Social Psychology, 61*(2), 195–202. https://doi.org/10.1037/0022-3514.61.2.195

Slovic, P. (2000). *The perception of risk*. Earthscan Publications.

Tversky, A., & Kahneman, D. (1973). Availability: A heuristic for judging frequency and probability. *Cognitive Psychology, 5*(2), 207–232. https://doi.org/10.1016/0010-0285(73)90033-9

Chapter 7
Negativity Bias. Germany and Laparoscopic Surgery

The Problem

Kurt Karl Stephan Semm (Bhattacharya, 2007) was a German gynecologist and professor of gynecology at Christian Albrecht University, located in Kiel, the most populous city in northern Germany and a major maritime center on the Baltic Sea. Although procedures assisted by optical instruments (such as liver biopsy) were already being performed at the time, Semm initially focused his work on the study of infertility and the use of endoscopic methods for diagnostic purposes (pelviscopy), expanding to laparoscopic gynecology. Together with other colleagues, he co-founded the German Society of Fertility and Sterility in 1958. However, there was significant resistance to the endoscopic approach in gynecology at the time, to the extent that, during one of his lectures on ovarian cyst resection, the slide projector was disconnected to prevent the presentation of "*unethical surgeries*" (Bhattacharya, 2007). Despite the rejection, motivated by the promise of the technique, Semm soon began performing therapeutic gynecological procedures, for which he invented several instruments, including the CO_2 insufflator and various coagulation and suturing devices. In 1970, he was appointed director of the Department of Gynecology and Obstetrics at the University of Kiel; however, the appointment required him to undergo a brain scan at the request of his colleagues, as "*only a person with brain damage would perform laparoscopic surgery*." Similarly, the German gynecological community referred to the technique as "*nonsense*" (Brown, 2005). Nevertheless, Semm persisted in his vision, and by 1980 he was already recognized as an authority in operative endoscopic gynecology.

On September 13, 1980, Semm performed the first incidental laparoscopic appendectomy in a patient with extensive pelvic endometriosis, and his experience was presented at a surgical meeting in 1981 (Mettler, 2003). Despite the patient's favorable recovery and absence of complications, Semm faced strong criticism, with the procedure being labeled as "*unethical*" and demands for the suspension of his medical license by Dr. Kurt Spohn, then president of the German Surgical Society (Pia Rieger,

A. Sanabria and C. Betancourt, *Cognitive Biases in Surgical Practice*,
https://doi.org/10.1007/978-3-032-20377-9_7

2017). Despite multiple attempts and rejections by prestigious journals such as the American Journal of Obstetrics and Gynecology, it was not until 1983 that Semm was able to publish his results, first in a local German journal (Semm, 1983a) and later in an international journal (Semm, 1983b). During these years, Semm persistently suggested to surgeons the possibility of exploring laparoscopic cholecystectomy, but was met with reluctance and ridicule by general surgeons, who disparagingly referred to it as "*keyhole surgery*" (Alkatout et al., 2021) and mockingly called him "*the chairman of the Magic Club*" (Litynski, 1998).

Despite all this, five years later, on September 12, 1985, Erich Mühe, a surgeon from Böblingen, a city in southern Germany, performed the first laparoscopic cholecystectomy using instruments designed by Semm. Mühe faced the same criticisms as Semm (Litynski, 1998) when he presented his experience with 94 patients in 1986, and the procedure was ridiculed as "*Mickey Mouse surgery.*" He was even sued in German courts for involuntary homicide when one of his patients died. Three years later, he was fully exonerated (Stern, 2013).

Among other arguments, opponents of laparoscopic surgery claimed that this alternative was more complicated, more time-consuming, required new instruments, did not allow visualization of the entire abdominal cavity, needed learning specific skills for intracorporeal knot tying, etc. (Fig. 7.1).

Despite all the resistance, the benefits of laparoscopic surgery became too evident to be denied. Gradually, doubts were transformed into certainties, and procedures

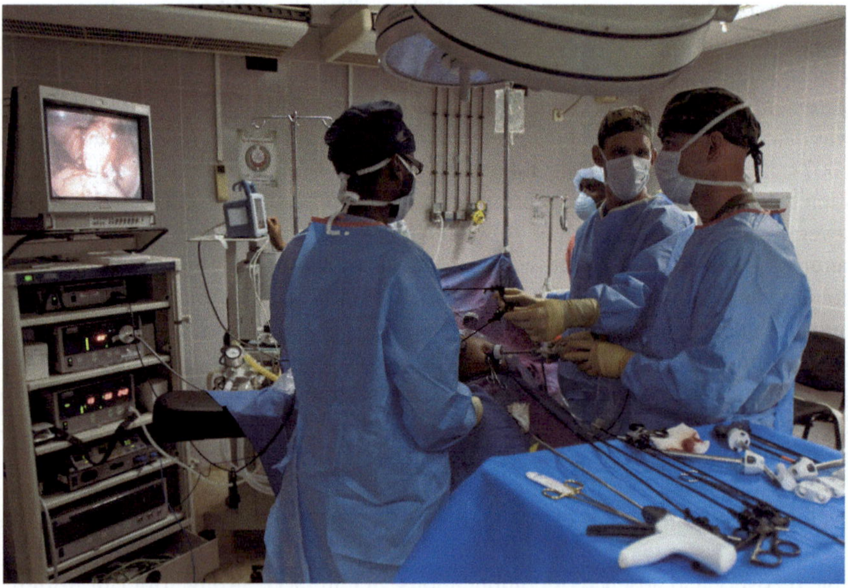

Fig. 7.1 Laparoscopic surgery (Public domain) https://ggia.berkeley.edu/ (File:US Navy 081117-N-7526R-568 Cmdr. Thomas Nelson and Lt. Robert Roadfuss discuss proper procedures while performing a laparoscopic cholecystectomy surgery.jpg)

using this approach became established, standardized, and disseminated throughout Germany and the rest of the world. In 1994, the same society that had requested the cancellation of his medical license awarded Semm the *Johannes-von-Mikulicz-Radecki—Georg-Kelling* prize for the creation and development of endoscopic surgery. Mühe was recognized as a pioneer in laparoscopic surgery by the German Society of Surgery in 1992.

Laparoscopic appendectomy and cholecystectomy are currently the gold standard for the management of surgical pathologies of the appendix and gallbladder. Training in these procedures is included in all general surgery programs worldwide. Laparoscopic instruments and techniques have advanced to such an extent that virtually all open abdominal procedures can now also be performed laparoscopically. The advantages of this minimally invasive approach are so significant that they have enabled this shift. In retrospect, it seems almost absurd and even ridiculous to think that these techniques and approaches were once criticized and rejected. Nevertheless, this was unfortunately the case. The question arises: How could this have happened? How could a novel technique, clearly beneficial for patients, have been so openly dismissed? To what extent can surgeons' fears hinder the acceptance of techniques and procedures that clearly improve upon those available at the time? The answer lies in negativity bias, one of the most prominent factors influencing our evaluation of everyday situations.

Definition

Given equal stimulus intensity, the activation of cognitive functions (attention, perception, memory, affect, behavior, and decision-making) is stronger, faster, and more enduring in response to a negative stimulus (dangerous, undesirable, or painful) than to a positive stimulus (desirable, beneficial, or pleasurable). In more colloquial terms, negative events are stronger, more prominent, and more persistent than positive events; therefore, humans are more attentive to them, devote more time to them, and assign them greater weight (Cacioppo et al., 2014). With regard to moral judgments, people use negative information much more than positive information to form an impression of someone (Vaish et al., 2008). This phenomenon is defined as negativity bias (Norris, 2021).

In addition to strong resistance to change, the situation described exemplifies the effect of negativity bias. Most critics and detractors focused on technical difficulties, complications, excessive costs, the need for "extra" training, and other potential negative outcomes, arguing that these made the introduction of laparoscopic surgery impossible. All of these were negative aspects of the new procedure, which were given greater weight and importance than the benefits, such as avoiding a larger incision, reducing the risk of postoperative evisceration and late incisional hernia, faster recovery of intestinal transit, decreased postoperative pain, and a faster return to daily activities. This led to unjustified attacks against the proposing surgeon and the technique itself, initially hindering the development and implementation of the minimally invasive surgical alternative in Germany, only for it to be reconsidered after being accepted in other countries. Today, both laparoscopic techniques, appendectomy and cholecystectomy, are considered standard management (Jaschinski et al., 2018).

History

There is a long history of the predominance of negative situations over positive ones in terms of value. The philosophical pessimism of Arthur Schopenhauer is a representative example, though not the only one of the impact of a negative and pessimistic worldview.

In 1971, Guido Peeters (Peeters, 1971) from the Laboratorium voor Experimentele Sociale Psychologie, University of Leuven, addressed the situation from the perspective of positivism bias and established the concept of positive-negative asymmetry. He specified that although positive events are more frequent in people's lives, humans attribute greater urgency to negative events, which, although less frequent, have more catastrophic consequences.

In their prospect theory, Kahneman and Tversky in 1979 described loss aversion as the greater psychological discomfort experienced in the face of a loss, compared to a gain of the same magnitude, thereby reinforcing the concept that negative events have a greater impact (Kahneman & Tversky, 1979).

In 1994, John Cacioppo and Gary Berntson from the Department of Psychology at Ohio State University (Cacioppo & Berntson, 1994) proposed that the evaluations of positivity and negativity are two separate functions which, through an internal balance, can determine the approach or avoidance of a given stimulus, within a model they called the *Model of Evaluative Space.* This explains why the same phenomenon can elicit different responses in both quality and magnitude. Their research demonstrated that the same stimulus produces faster, stronger, and more sustained responses in the negative domain compared to the positive (Norris, 2021).

By 2001, Paul Rozin and Edward Poyzman from the Department of Psychology and the Solomon Asch Center for the Study of Ethnopolitical Conflict at the University of Pennsylvania (Rozin & Royzman, 2001) compiled previous evidence and provided a theoretical framework for the bias, outlining its four constitutive elements that are accepted today: *negative potency* (negative information is more powerful and prominent), *greater steepness of negative gradients* (negative information increases more rapidly than positive), *negativity dominance* (negative information has a greater impact than positive), and *negative differentiation* (negative information is richer in gradation than positive).

Some authors have proposed that negativity bias has an adaptive explanation within evolution, where functions aimed at improving survival and maintaining reproduction are prioritized. In these terms, negative events (such as accidents or death) tend to impact survival to a greater extent than positive events (Cacioppo et al., 2014) and, moreover, are more difficult to reverse once they have occurred. In this regard, there is evidence that by 12 months of age, children already exhibit a clear negativity bias (Vaish et al., 2008). Physiologically, it has been shown that gustatory sensitivity to bitter foods (which are often harmful to health) is much greater than to sweet foods. Other examples include the greater ease of locating areas in space where negative stimuli are present. However, there is also evidence indicating that negativity bias decreases with age (Mather & Carstensen, 2005).

Impact

Due to increased sensitivity to negative stimuli, greater perception of their magnitude, and the longer duration of their effects, the negativity bias produces multiple effects in everyday life. Among the most significant are:

At the Personal Level

1. **Excessive focus on negative events:** In daily interactions, negative events (errors, complications) are more frequently highlighted than positive ones (successes, recovery). Such emphasis may be perceived as unwarranted criticism or aggressive attitudes, which can disrupt personal relationships and institutional work dynamics.
2. **Aversion to acknowledging negative events and their effects:** Describing negative events is often associated with feelings such as shame or incompetence and is accompanied by some form of blame and/or punishment. This effect occurs during medical training and persists through the highest levels of specialization (with an emphasis on complications and errors in medical education). (Haizlip et al., 2012) This can create for example a culture of not reporting adverse events, concealing them when they occur, or failing to acknowledge them when they are demonstrated.
3. **Cognitive distortions:** Negativity bias can promote the emergence of cognitive distortions such as black-and-white thinking (seeing things as either bad or good, with no shades of gray), overgeneralization (paying greater attention to infrequent negative events may lead to the belief that everything is negative), magnification (allocating more importance to a negative event than it actually warrants), and false prediction (assuming that the occurrence of a negative event predicts a negative trajectory and outcome).

At the Collective Level

1. **Commitment to Competitiveness:** Working groups may be affected by an excessive focus on negative aspects (e.g., delays in the initiation of procedures, prolonged waiting times) and minimal attention to positive aspects (e.g., customer satisfaction, efficient use of resources). This can lead to a reactive attitude, lack of

collaboration, and reduced engagement. Additionally, it may decrease creativity and slow down innovation.

2. **Motivational function:** Since negativity bias is associated with loss aversion bias, it can be used as a motivator to encourage behavior change. Leveraging the potential loss of an already earned incentive can serve as a motivator for behavioral modification. For example, instead of awarding bonuses at the end of a period as a reward for performance (such as punctuality or meeting deadlines), awards can be given at the beginning, with deductions made at the end of the period based on actual performance (Mather & Carstensen, 2005).

Examples in Medical and Surgical Practice

Unfortunately, negative outcomes are an inescapable part of medical practice. Thus, the effects of negativity bias in the professional practice of physicians and surgeons are multiple and varied. Among these, the following can be mentioned:

1. **Neglect of negative outcomes:** Such as underreporting or failure to report complications and adverse events related to surgery, which are neither disclosed nor analyzed due to their association with humiliating, disqualifying, or punitive attitudes (Elwy et al., 2016).
2. **Diagnostic Errors:** When Emphasis is placed on evaluating patients to rule out negative findings, which are then given greater weight in the context of disease. Thus, medical semiology is grounded in the paradigm of seeking and identifying negative signs (e.g., arrhythmias instead of a regular pulse) and symptoms (e.g., drowsiness instead of wakefulness). When such findings are detected, they are given increased significance in the diagnostic context. For example, "*every case of right lower abdominal pain is considered appendicitis until proven otherwise.*"
3. **Non-constructive evaluations by colleagues or supervising staff:** Performance assessment and training progress are often focused on error avoidance rather than on enhancing skills and competencies. Thus, the evaluation of physicians, undergraduate and postgraduate students centers on the number of inadequately performed steps rather than on those performed correctly (Ebertz et al., 2019). Institutional certification and monitoring mechanisms are based on the percentage of adverse events or complications, rather than on effectiveness. When commenting on a colleague's performance, negative aspects (complications) are usually highlighted, while positive outcomes (recovery) are often overlooked (Niu et al., 2020).
4. **Catastrophic view of professional practice:** Since negative events tend to persist over time, their recollection can alter the surgeon's attitude toward the practice of the profession. In response to a negative event, the surgeon may adopt a defensive approach in diagnostic testing (*overdiagnosis*) or in performing procedures (*overtreatment*). This attitude, along with the feelings associated with the negative event, may persist for extended periods, develop into fear or a sense of

inadequacy, and even contribute to the onset of disorders such as depression or anxiety.

5. **Poorly oriented meetings:** Multidisciplinary meetings focused on negative aspects of surgery, such as "*complications*" meetings, "*adverse events*" reviews, "*performance*" evaluations, etc. It is rare to find meetings on "*success*" or "*best practices.*"

How to Prevent Bias

Although it is clear that surgical culture cannot be separated from the predominance of negative events, some of the strategies suggested to mitigate the effect of negativity bias include:

1. **Balance the presentation of positive and negative events:** In meetings involving performance or skills evaluation, begin with the negative events, using neutral language, and conclude with the positive outcomes. This approach aligns with the principle that the last observation tends to remain longer in the mind of the person being evaluated. In this regard, evidence suggests that balancing the impact of a single negative event requires between four and nine positive events.
2. **Focus the discussion of adverse events on contextual factors rather than the individual:** Questions that begin with how or why should take precedence over those that begin with who or when. This approach allows the adverse event to be viewed as a learning opportunity, removing the deleterious effects of shame or perceived incompetence.
3. **Facilitate positive framing:** In situations where the frequency of negative events is traditionally assessed, it is possible to shift the framing toward demonstrating the frequency of positive events. For example, when evaluating the frequency of surgical wound infection, instead of reporting the percentage of occurrence, the percentage of absence can be used.
4. **Mindfulness training:** Negativity bias predicts that negative events are perceived as stronger and more enduring than positive ones, even in the face of clear evidence that the latter are equal to or even better than the former. Mindfulness, by focusing attention, enables a more balanced assessment of different events and reduces rumination on negative experiences (Kiken Shook, 2011).
5. **Avoid information sources that exploit negativity bias, such as social media:** These platforms commercially or politically exploit advertising based on fear, guilt, or urgency, all negative events. Limiting exposure to such information sources allows for a more balanced analysis of different events.
6. **Keeping a "*gratitude*" journal:** Institutions focused on promoting healthy lifestyle habits recommend keeping a "*gratitude*" journal, which can be understood as a record of positive events aimed at counteracting the greater influence of negative events in daily life. This practice can be applied to professional settings by recording patients who have improved or recovered (UC Berkeley, 2025).

References

Alkatout, I., Mechler, U., Mettler, L., Pape, J., Maass, N., Biebl, M., Gitas, G., Lagana, A. S., & Freytag, D. (2021). The development of laparoscopy—A historical overview. *Frontiers in Surgery, 8*, 799442. https://doi.org/10.3389/fsurg.2021.799442

Bhattacharya, K. (2007). Kurt Semm: A laparoscopic crusader. *The Journal of Minimal Access Surgery, 3*(1), 35–36. https://doi.org/10.4103/0972-9941.30686

Brown, S. (2005). *ESHRE. The first 21 years* (1st ed.). European Society of Human Reproduction and Embryology (ESHRE). https://www.eshre.eu/Home/About-us/History

Cacioppo, J. T., & Berntson, G. G. (1994). Relationship between attitudes and evaluative space: A critical review, with emphasis on the separability of positive and negative substrates. *Psychological Bulletin, 115*(3), 401–423. https://doi.org/10.1037/0033-2909.115.3.401

Cacioppo, J. T., Cacioppo, S., & Gollan, J. K. (2014). The negativity bias: Conceptualization, quantification, and individual differences. *The Behavioral and Brain Sciences, 37*(3), 309–310. https://doi.org/10.1017/S0140525X13002537

Ebertz, D. P., Hong, H. Y., Kafai, N. M., Evie, H. P., & Salles, A. (2019). Written evaluations of surgical residents: Are they biased? *Journal of the American College of Surgeons, 229*(4, Supplement 1), S254. https://doi.org/10.1016/j.jamcollsurg.2019.08.558

Elwy, A. R., Itani, K. M., Bokhour, B. G., Mueller, N. M., Glickman, M. E., Zhao, S., Rosen, A. K., Lynge, D., Perkal, M., Brotschi, E. A., Sanchez, V. M., & Gallagher, T. H. (2016). Surgeons' disclosures of clinical adverse events. *JAMA Surgery, 151*(11), 1015–1021. https://doi.org/10.1001/jamasurg.2016.1787

Haizlip, J., May, N., Schorling, J., Williams, A., & Plews-Ogan, M. (2012). Perspective: The negativity bias, medical education, and the culture of academic medicine: Why culture change is hard. *Academic Medicine, 87*(9), 1205–1209. https://doi.org/10.1097/ACM.0b013e3182628f03

Jaschinski, T., Mosch, C. G., Eikermann, M., Neugebauer, E. A., & Sauerland, S. (2018). Laparoscopic versus open surgery for suspected appendicitis. *Cochrane Database of Systematic Reviews, 11*(11), CD001546. https://doi.org/10.1002/14651858.CD001546.pub4

Kahneman, D., & Tversky, A. (1979). Prospect theory: An analysis of decision under risk. *Econometrica, 47*(2), 263–291. https://doi.org/10.2307/1914185

Kiken, L. G., & Shook, N. J. (2011). Looking up: Mindfulness increases positive judgments and reduces negativity bias. Sage Publications. https://doi.org/10.1177/1948550610396585

Litynski, G. S. (1998). Kurt Semm and the fight against skepticism: Endoscopic hemostasis, laparoscopic appendectomy, and Semm's impact on the "laparoscopic revolution". *JSLS, 2*(3), 309–313.

Mather, M., & Carstensen, L. L. (2005). Aging and motivated cognition: The positivity effect in attention and memory. *Trends in Cognitive Sciences, 9*(10), 496–502. https://doi.org/10.1016/j.tics.2005.08.005

Mettler, L. (2003). Historical profile of Kurt Karl Stephan Semm, born march 23, 1927 in Munich, Germany, resident of Tucson, Arizona, USA since 1996. *Jsls, 7*(3), 185–188.

Niu, M., Gaerth, M., & Kraus, F. (2020). *Share my failure, not my success: How people make ubiquity judgments based on past events*. European Marketing Academy.

Norris, C. J. (2021). The negativity bias, revisited: Evidence from neuroscience measures and an individual differences approach. *Social Neuroscience, 16*(1), 68–82. https://doi.org/10.1080/17470919.2019.1696225

Peeters, G. (1971). The positive-negative asymmetry: On cognitive consistency and positivity bias. *European Journal of Social Psychology, 1*(4), 455–474. https://doi.org/10.1002/ejsp.2420010405

Pia Rieger, C. (2017). *The negative appendectomy rate in a southern German Center with two locations—Histopathological evaluation over a one-year period in 2014* Ludwig Maximilian University of Munich]. Augsburg. Chrome-extension: //efaidnbmnnnibpcajpcglclefindmkaj/ https://edoc.ub.uni-muenchen.de/21715/1/Rieger_Carmen_Pia.pdf

Rozin, P., & Royzman, E. B. (2001). Negativity bias, negativity dominance, and contagion. *Personality and Social Psychology Review, 5*(4), 296–320. https://doi.org/10.1207/S15327957PSPR0504_2

Semm, K. (1983a). The endoscopic appendectomy. *Gynecology Practice, 7*, 131–140.

Semm, K. (1983b). Endoscopic appendectomy. *Endoscopy, 15*(2), 59–64. https://doi.org/10.1055/s-2007-1021466

Stern, V. (2013). The first lap Chole in Europe: A 'criminal' is vindicated. *General Surgery News*. https://www.generalsurgerynews.com/In-the-News/Article/06-13/The-first-Lap-Chole-in-Europe-A-%E2%80%98Criminal%E2%80%99-Is-Vindicated/23368

UC Berkeley. (2025). Greater good science center. *Science-based practice for a meaningful life.* Retrieved from October 23, 2025, https://ggia.berkeley.edu/

Vaish, A., Grossmann, T., & Woodward, A. (2008). Not all emotions are created equal: The negativity bias in social-emotional development. *Psychological Bulletin, 134*(3), 383–403. https://doi.org/10.1037/0033-2909.134.3.383

Chapter 8
Illusory Correlation: Angina and Ligation of the Internal Mammary Artery

The Problem

Claude Beck, an American cardiac surgeon who spent his entire career at Case Western Reserve University and the Cleveland Clinic, was the first to propose improving cardiac vascular flow as a method to treat myocardial ischemia (Theruvath & Ikonomidis, 2015). Building on this idea, Davide Fieschi (Negro et al., 2014), an Italian surgeon practicing in Bergamo, proposed in 1939 a surgical technique for the treatment of angina pectoris. His approach was based on the pathophysiological rationale that bilateral ligation of the internal mammary artery (Fig. 8.1) would redirect more blood flow to vessels near the heart, thereby increasing blood supply to the coronary arteries and alleviating symptoms. He published his initial experience in 1942 with a single patient followed for two years, reporting remarkable improvement. However, he was imprisoned by the fascist regime, and his work was forgotten for several years.

In October 1955, three physicians from the Department of Surgery at the University of Parma (Mario Battezzati, Alberto Tagliaferro, and G. De Marchi) published a study in the Italian journal *Minerva Medica*, reporting two additional cases of patients with remarkable responses to their angina. By 1959, they had reported the astonishing number of 304 patients treated with this method, with symptom improvement observed in 94% of cases and electrocardiogram changes in 64% (Battezzati et al., 1959). With these extraordinary results, the alternative quickly spread throughout Italy.

Simultaneously, Robert P. Glover and Roderick Kitchell (Glover et al., 1958; Kitchell et al., 1958), who led a group in Philadelphia, published two articles in June of 1958 that altered the course of efforts to improve cardiac circulation. They presented the results of animal experiments confirming a connection between the mammary arteries and the coronary arteries, as well as outcomes from 92 patients who underwent the procedure (50 of whom were followed for up to 6 months). Improvement in symptoms and electrocardiogram findings occurred in 64% and

A. Sanabria and C. Betancourt, *Cognitive Biases in Surgical Practice*,
https://doi.org/10.1007/978-3-032-20377-9_8

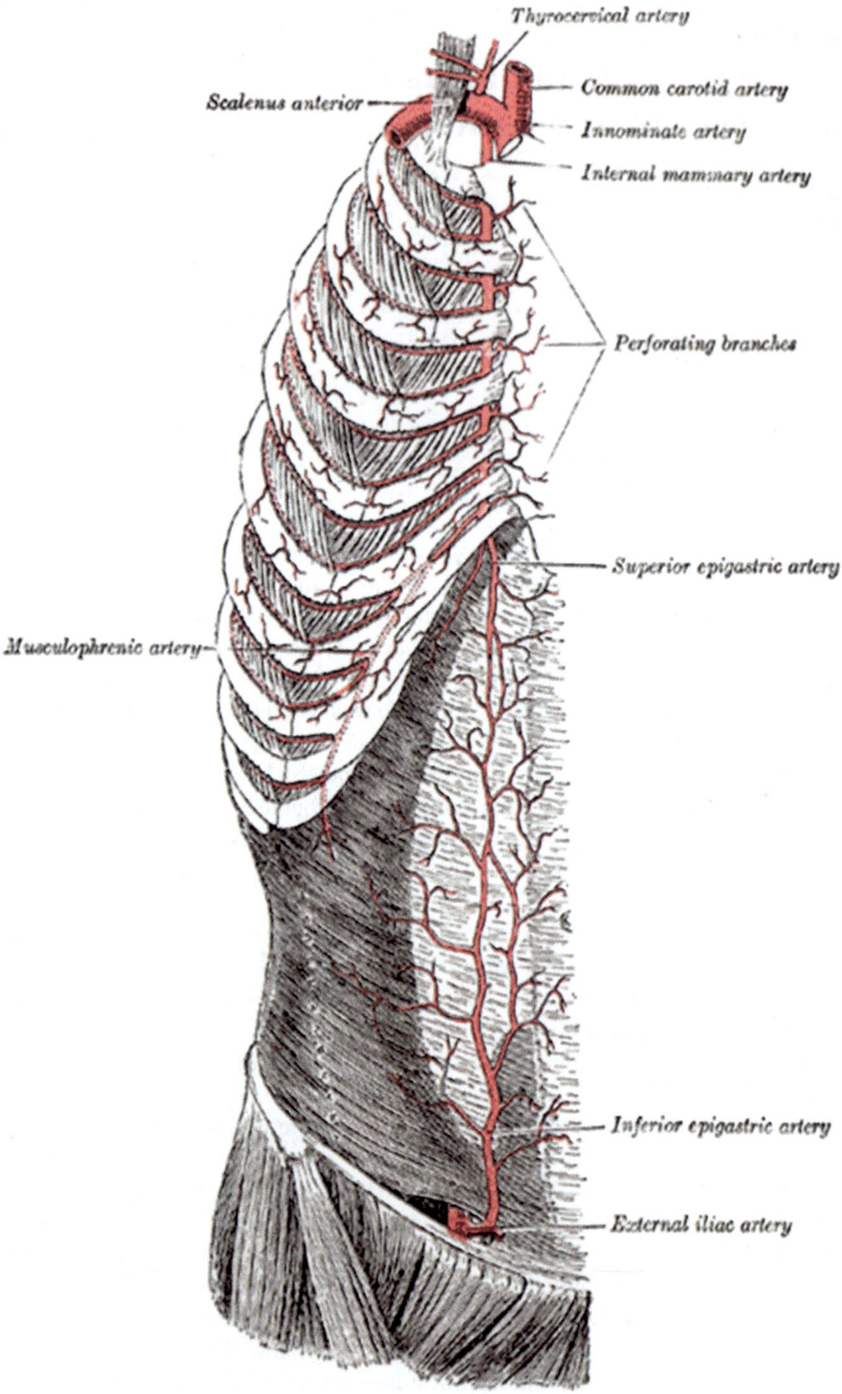

Fig. 8.1 Internal mammary artery (public domain) Henry Vandyke Carter

43% of patients, respectively. These results were reported in the popular press in 1957 by John D. Ratcliff, a prolific science journalist who wrote for Reader's Digest (Ratcliff, 1957). In his article, he echoed the findings of Battezzati and Glover. The news quickly spread, and many European and American centers adopted the technique.

Nevertheless, doubts quickly arose. Several surgeons criticized the findings and attempted to demonstrate the lack of effectiveness of the intervention (Adams, 1958; Fish et al., 1958). In 1959, Rudolph Fremont, Robert Klopstock, and Paul Glass from the Brooklyn Veterans Administration Hospital and the State University of New York (Fremont et al., 1959) were the first to use "*sham surgery*" to evaluate the effectiveness of this intervention. In this procedure, they performed a thoracic incision similar to that of mammary artery ligation, but without tying off the vessels. In a study with a small sample size, they were unable to reproduce the dramatic findings of previous studies. However, they suggested that the psychological component in patients eager for improvement could impact symptoms, and that the intervention might not have a real effect on the disease. They also suggested that the evaluators may not have been strict enough in assessing the symptoms. On May 28, 1959, nearly 20 years after Fieschi's initial proposal and after a significant number of patients had undergone surgery, Leonard Cobb and his collaborators at the University of Washington (Cobb et al., 1959), using Fremont's sham or placebo surgery approach, designed a randomized clinical trial with 17 patients, demonstrating the absence of effect of bilateral mammary artery ligation in improving angina symptoms. Dimond and colleagues confirmed these findings in 1960 (Dimond et al., 1960). Glover promptly accepted the results that contradicted his initial findings (Glover et al., 1960), and Battezzati put up a brief resistance, but soon ceased to defend the idea. Bilateral mammary artery ligation was abandoned as a treatment, but it laid the groundwork for the use of mammary circulation in cardiac revascularization that was developed later.

Today, the idea that ligating an artery in the thoracic wall could help improve myocardial perfusion seems absurd, if not laughable. Nevertheless, this procedure was performed for more than 20 years in a considerable number of patients. The question that arises is how this could have happened. How could a personal experience in an extremely limited group of patients have such widespread impact? How could a case series without a control group be disseminated and promoted as a panacea for myocardial ischemia? Even more concerning, how could so many professionals and patients accept it when there was no logical basis for the procedure? The answer lies in illusory correlation, one of the cognitive biases that most strongly influences how we establish associations and causal relationships.

Definition

Contingency is defined as the possibility of a relationship between events. In psychology, it refers to the causal, temporal, and probabilistic relationship between two or more events, involving an exposure and an outcome. If contingency exists, the two events are closely related, and it can be expected that one is the consequence of the other. When there is no contingency, the two events occur randomly, independently of each other. In this context, illusory correlation arises when one believes there is a relationship between two events when, in fact, none exists.

This cognitive bias involves perceiving relationships that do not actually exist between variables (people, events, or behaviors) simply because they occur simultaneously or sequentially. Examples include stereotypes that associate certain characteristics with membership in a specific group, with illusory correlation serving as one of the foundations for biases related to gender, age, race, religion, and politics. It also provides a coherent explanation for superstitions, folklore, and magical beliefs.

Although the negative effects of bias are undeniable, there are situations where its presence can be beneficial, such as when it is used to promote healthy behaviors (certain natural diets and improved sexual functioning) or moral behaviors (helping someone today will lead to receiving help from others in the future).

In the case of internal mammary artery ligation, a few cases observed by surgeons eager to find a solution to a problem, presenting evidence in favor of a procedure that appeared convincing, effective, and simple to perform; put a surgical intervention in motion. The intervention and the apparent improvement in symptoms, a simple and direct causal relationship, suggested that the procedure could be beneficial. However, in those initial reports, the authors and other professionals who adopted the technique did not question the absence of a control group to allow for comparison of results and to rule out other causes; they did not ask why there was such an immediate resolution of symptoms; they did not seek to confirm the mechanisms that could explain such dramatic success (the studies that validated the animal experiments failed to find the so-called "*anastomoses*" between the cardiac and internal mammary circulations); nor did they address the inconsistency between subjective outcome measures (improvement in pain and symptoms) and objective measurements (electrocardiogram changes). At the end, many patients underwent a completely useless surgery for the intended purpose.

History

The issue of erroneous associations has been explored in philosophy since the Renaissance. David Hume, a Scottish philosopher, provided a framework for its study by proposing *Hume's Challenge to Reason.*

In 1967, Loren James Chapman, a professor at Southern Illinois University, published an article in which he described the "*systematic error of reporting a correlation that is not supported by objective facts*," calling it illusory correlation (Chapman, 1967). In his definition, Chapman identified three variant types of this bias: when there is no correlation at all, when a correlation exists but is weaker than perceived by the subject, and when the correlation exists but in the opposite direction to that proposed by the subject. The original study exposed subjects to pairs of words that were similar in length or meaning and demonstrated that experimental subjects tended to create nonexistent associations between these words. That same year, together with his colleague and wife Jean Paulsen Chapman, he published a study (Chapman & Chapman, 1967) demonstrating the existence of the illusory correlation bias by testing the results of psychodynamic assessments such as the Draw-a-Person Test (DAP) and, subsequently in 1969, the Rorschach test (Chapman & Chapman, 1969). They showed that the relationship between certain personal traits and test results was the product of associations unsupported by the data, and that both clinicians and laypeople were equally susceptible to this error.

In 1976, David Hamilton and Robert Gifford (Hamilton & Gifford, 1976), then psychologists at Yale University, extended the original proposal to the study of stereotypes, demonstrating that people form correlations between certain characteristics (physical, geographical, etc.) and behaviors in a random manner, which are later accepted as real. Since infrequent stimuli or events receive more attention than frequent ones, due to their greater availability, nonexistent associations are created when they appear together (distinctiveness-based illusory correlation). More recently, Klaus Fiedler and Peter Freytag from the University of Heidelberg (Fiedler et al., 2009) proposed that, rather than a memory failure, illusory correlation is due to an adaptive mechanism that seeks to extract information from events that occur frequently and for which there is no information available to refute this co-occurrence (information loss account).

Impact

Illusory correlation can become a decisive factor in people's lives and influence daily decision-making, as it creates a nonexistent connection between factors that can alter behavior.

At the Personal Level

1. **Reinforcement of nonexistent causal relationships.** When there is a high expectation of association between two variables, it has been shown that the illusory correlation will be stronger. For example, if one believes that traffic is worse in a particular city, it is likely that being caught in a traffic jam will reinforce this perceived correlation.
2. **Creation and maintenance of stereotypes.** When stereotypes exist, illusory correlation is likely to reinforce them and may even escalate them to the level of prejudice or discrimination, such as when certain behaviors are associated with people from specific geographic areas and this association appears to be confirmed by paying more attention to these two characteristics than to all others.

At the Collective Level

1. **Increase in polarization.** The media (radio, television, newspapers, and social networks) tend to create illusory correlations (associations between the frequency

of certain behaviors and specific neighborhoods in a city) or reinforce existing ones (cases of corruption associated with certain professions), thereby increasing discrimination and polarization.

2. **Creation of conspiracy theories.** The emergence and strengthening of conspiracy theories are rooted in illusory correlation, which generates nonexistent associations and patterns between events. For example, linking historical phenomena to individual decisions without considering the broader context of the era.
3. **Perpetuation of inequalities.** The false association between personality traits and physical characteristics can sustain or deepen inequalities or behaviors in certain environments, such as when someone is more readily evaluated or hired based on their clothing or manner of speaking. A similar phenomenon occurs in marketing, where the use of products is associated with certain pleasurable sensations.
4. **Formation of irrational behaviors.** Illusory correlation can also produce or explain irrational behaviors such as rituals and superstitions (for example, walking around the block on New Year's Eve is believed to promote long-distance travel during the year).
5. **Use of discriminatory language.** The mere labeling of a characteristic or behavior can create illusory correlations. An uncommon or emotionally charged name may become associated with another feature sharing similar attributes (for instance, the group "W," where "W" is an infrequent letter in the alphabet, ends up being linked to an undesirable condition).

Examples in Medical and Surgical Practice

The practice of medicine and surgery, more than most professions, involves the continual establishment of associations and causal relationships. Therefore, it is to be expected that the effects of illusory correlation are numerous and varied. Among the most significant are:

1. **Erroneous clinical decision-making:** Decision-making in surgery is based on the results of clinical studies that assess the risk of exposure leading to an outcome and the effectiveness of an intervention in modifying a disease. It is well known that retrospective observational studies (the most common study design in medical publications) carry a high risk of selection bias and, therefore, of attributing nonexistent causal relationships. This explains why some observational studies suggest associations that are later refuted by studies with greater methodological rigor. Nevertheless, physicians often adopt the conclusions of these lower-quality studies because they are the most prevalent in literature (Benson & Hartz, 2000).
2. **Diagnosis and treatment based on patient stereotypes:** When treating a certain group of patients, surgeons may be influenced by stereotypes that are part of the hidden curriculum taught in medical schools. For example, there are stereotypes

about patients with certain conditions (e.g., obesity) regarding their adherence to treatments (e.g., dietary or physical activity modifications), which can lead to the premature or unnecessary offering of surgical interventions (Madey & Ondrus, 1999).

3. **False causal association:** Erroneously believing that an exposure is linked to a particular outcome can lead to the creation of entirely incorrect causal relationships. For instance, there is information suggesting a relationship between radiation exposure and the development of certain malignant tumors, such as thyroid cancer. When the Chernobyl accident occurred in 1986, many new cases of thyroid tumors in Europe were attributed to radiation exposure from the nuclear accident. Some experts suggested that, although a causal relationship existed, it was not of the magnitude that was reported. When the Fukushima accident occurred in 2011, scientists were aware of this possibility. Subsequent studies showed that, while there was a relationship between radiation and thyroid cancer incidence, the magnitude was not as high, and other factors, such as increased screening, helped explain the rise in incidence (Ohtsuru et al., 2019).
4. **Biased performance evaluation:** The surgeon's role encompasses clinical, administrative, and medical education activities. As one of the elements highlighting stereotypes, illusory correlation can affect how surgeons evaluate the performance of their team members and the students under their supervision. For example, evidence shows that race, socioeconomic status, gender, language, and other factors influence evaluations made for professional or academic purposes. In the USA, Black, Asian, and international students tend to receive lower performance ratings compared to White, American, and native English-speaking students (Bandyopadhyay et al., 2022).
5. **Irrational behaviors:** By generating false cause and effect, illusory correlation also gives rise to a range of bizarre and absurd behaviors. For example, during the COVID-19 pandemic, many physicians proposed the use of agents such as acetic acid or vodka for handwashing, boxes to contain aerosols during intubation, or chloroquine or ivermectin as methods to prevent infection, all based on false causalities (Rubin, 2022).

How to Avoid Falling into Bias

1. **Foster critical thinking:** Assessing the causal relationship between a given exposure or intervention and an outcome is one of the foundations of medicine and surgery. However, studies have shown that most physicians, like other human beings, are highly susceptible to the illusory correlation bias. Training based on scientific knowledge helps reduce the impact of this bias. Training alternatives that incorporate critical thinking tools (such as alternative thinking, lateral thinking, and epidemiology) taught from an early stage are valuable resources. They can even serve as debiasing strategies when applied in environments with a high prevalence of bias (Matute et al., 2015).
2. **Encourage diverse perspectives:** Since many illusory correlations are embedded in the mindset of surgeons, measures to mitigate their effect can be

beneficial. Personal exposure to members of minority groups, who are often the subjects of illusory correlations, and the presentation of a greater amount of accurate information have proven useful. Similarly, if there is a perception that a particular surgical procedure is associated with more adverse events, presenting multiple advocates demonstrating that the frequency of such events is similar across procedures can reduce bias (Murphy et al., 2011).

3. **Learning to focus on empirical evidence:** In settings such as multidisciplinary meetings where there is a high risk of illusory correlation (e.g., the perceived relationship between certain symptoms and a diagnosis, or between a specific therapeutic approach and an expected outcome), providing objective data (such as a table showing the frequency of symptoms and their association with the diagnosis, or the frequency of a particular treatment and its outcomes) before making a judgment can reduce the impact of bias (Berndsen et al., 1996).
4. **Recognize susceptibility to bias:** Since this bias is so pervasive, efforts to make it visible and to help decision-makers understand their own susceptibility are highly relevant (Stroessner & Plaks, 2001). Exercises such as emphasizing a more reasoned approach ("*listen carefully to the following arguments*") or a more distinctive one ("*before forming an opinion, consider the existing differences and similarities*") prior to making a judgment have proven useful. The same applies to motivation. If there is a personal interest involved in the evaluation of variable occurrence, it is likely that illusory correlation will come into play. Mechanisms that make the effect of this personal motivation explicit ("*consider whether you have a conflict of interest*") can help reduce the impact of the bias.
5. **Blinding the decision-making process:** As has been observed, stereotypes depend on variables that people associate with certain outcomes or behaviors. One way to prevent these variables from influencing decisions is simply to disregard them. When making a diagnosis or offering treatment, omitting certain data can help ensure a more objective decision-making process. For example, omitting family history in cases of tumors where no such relationship has been demonstrated may help ensure that this factor does not erroneously influence the decision (Klein, 2005).

References

Adams, R. (1958). Internal mammary artery ligation for coronary insufficiency; An evaluation. *The New England Journal of Medicine, 258*(3), 113–115. https://doi.org/10.1056/NEJM195801162580302

Bandyopadhyay, S., Boylan, C. T., Baho, Y. G., Casey, A., Asif, A., Khalil, H., Badwi, N., & Patel, R. (2022). Ethnicity-related stereotypes and their impacts on medical students: A critical narrative review of health professions education literature. *Medical Teacher, 44*(9), 986–996. https://doi.org/10.1080/0142159X.2022.2051464

Battezzati, M., Tagliaferro, A., & Cattaneo, A. D. (1959). Clinical evaluation of bilateral internal mammary artery ligation as a treatment for coronary heart disease. *The American Journal of Cardiology, 4*(2), 180–183. https://doi.org/10.1016/0002-9149(59)90245-0

Benson, K., & Hartz, A. J. (2000). A comparison of observational studies and randomized, controlled trials. *The New England Journal of Medicine, 342*(25), 1878–1886. https://doi.org/10.1056/NEJM200006223422506

Berndsen, M., van der Pligt, J., Spears, R., & McGarty, C. (1996). *Expectation-based and data-based illusory correlation: The effects of confirming versus disconfirming evidence.* Wiley. https://doi.org/10.1002/(SICI)1099-0992(199611)

Chapman, L. J. (1967). Illusory correlation in observational report. *Journal of Verbal Learning & Verbal Behavior, 6*(1), 151–155. https://doi.org/10.1016/S0022-5371(67)80066-5

Chapman, L. J., & Chapman, J. P. (1967). *Genesis of popular but erroneous psychodiagnostic observations.* American Psychological Association. https://doi.org/10.1037/h0024670

Chapman, L. J., & Chapman, J. P. (1969). Illusory correlation as an obstacle to the use of valid psychodiagnostic indicators. *Journal of Abnormal Psychology, 74*(3), 271–280. https://doi.org/10.1037/h0027592

Cobb, L. A., Thomas, G. I., Dillard, D. H., Merendino, K. A., & Bruce, R. A. (1959). An evaluation of internal mammary artery ligation using a double-blind technique. *The New England Journal of Medicine, 260*(22), 1115–1118. https://doi.org/10.1056/NEJM195905282602204

Dimond, E. G., Kittle, C. F., & Crockett, J. E. (1960). Comparison of internal mammary artery ligation and sham operation for angina pectoris. *The American Journal of Cardiology, 5*, 483–486. https://doi.org/10.1016/0002-9149(60)90105-3

Fiedler, K., Freytag, P., & Meiser, T. (2009). Pseudocontingencies: An integrative account of an intriguing cognitive illusion. *Psychological Review, 116*, 187–206. https://doi.org/10.1037/a0014480

Fish, R. G., Crymes, T. P., & Lovell, M. G. (1958). Internal mammary artery ligation for angina pectoris; its failure to produce relief. *The New England Journal of Medicine, 259*(9), 418–420. https://doi.org/10.1056/NEJM195808282590903

Fremont, R. E., Klopstock, R., & Glass, P. (1959). Controlled studies on the efficacy of bilateral internal mammary artery ligation in patients with angina pectoris. *Angiology, 10*(1), 20–27. https://doi.org/10.1177/000331975901000103

Glover, R. P., Kitchell, J. R., Davila, J. C., & Barkley, H. T., Jr. (1960). Bilateral ligation of the internal mammary artery in the treatment of angina pectoris. Experimental and clinical results. *The American Journal of Cardiology, 6*, 937–945. https://doi.org/10.1016/0002-9149(60)90295-2

Glover, R. P., Kitchell, J. R., Kyle, R. H., Davila, J. C., & Trout, R. G. (1958). Experiences with myocardial revascularization by division of the internal mammary arteries. *Diseases of the Chest, 33*(6), 637–657. https://doi.org/10.1378/chest.33.6.637

Hamilton, D. L., & Gifford, R. K. (1976). *Illusory correlation in interpersonal perception: A cognitive basis of stereotypic judgments.* Elsevier. https://doi.org/10.1016/S0022-1031(76)80006-6

Kitchell, J. R., Glover, R. P., & Kyle, R. H. (1958). Bilateral internal mammary artery ligation for angina pectoris; preliminary clinical considerations. *The American Journal of Cardiology, 1*(1), 46–50. https://doi.org/10.1016/0002-9149(58)90074-2

Klein, J. G. (2005). Five pitfalls in decisions about diagnosis and prescribing. *BMJ, 330*(7494), 781–783. https://doi.org/10.1136/bmj.330.7494.781

Madey, S. F., & Ondrus, S. A. (1999). Illusory correlations in perceptions of noncooperative behaviors among obese and hypertensive patients. *Journal of Applied Social Psychology, 29*(6), 1200–1217. https://doi.org/10.1111/j.1559-1816.1999.tb02036.x

Matute, H., Blanco, F., Yarritu, I., Diaz-Lago, M., Vadillo, M. A., & Barberia, I. (2015). Illusions of causality: How they bias our everyday thinking and how they could be reduced. *Frontiers in Psychology, 6*, 888. https://doi.org/10.3389/fpsyg.2015.00888

Murphy, R. A., Schmeer, S., Vallee-Tourangeau, F., Mondragon, E., & Hilton, D. (2011). Making the illusory correlation effect appear and then disappear: The effects of increased learning. *Q J Exp Psychol (Hove), 64*(1), 24–40. https://doi.org/10.1080/17470218.2010.493615

Negro, P., Gossetti, F., Ceci, F., Manto, O., & D'Amore, L. (2014). Davide Fieschi: A pioneer of plug repair in groin hernia surgery. *Hernia, 18*(6), 919–923. https://doi.org/10.1007/s10029-013-1136-1

Ohtsuru, A., Midorikawa, S., Ohira, T., Suzuki, S., Takahashi, H., Murakami, M., Shimura, H., Matsuzuka, T., Yasumura, S., Suzuki, S. I., Yokoya, S., Hashimoto, Y., Sakai, A., Ohto, H., Yamashita, S., Tanigawa, K., & Kamiya, K. (2019). Incidence of thyroid cancer among children and young adults in Fukushima, Japan, screened with 2 rounds of ultrasonography within 5 years of the 2011 Fukushima Daiichi nuclear Power Station accident. *JAMA Otolaryngology. Head & Neck Surgery, 145*(1), 4–11. https://doi.org/10.1001/jamaoto.2018.3121

Ratcliff, J. (1957). New surgery for ailing hearts. *The Reader's Digest, 71*, 70–73.

Rubin, R. (2022). When physicians spread unscientific information about COVID-19. *JAMA, 327*(10), 904–906. https://doi.org/10.1001/jama.2022.1083

Stroessner, S. J., & Plaks, J. E. (2001). *Illusory correlation and stereotype formation: Tracing the arc of research over a quarter century*. Lawrence Erlbaum associates publishers.

Theruvath, T. P., & Ikonomidis, J. S. (2015). Historical perspectives of the American association for thoracic surgery: Claude S. Beck (1894–1971). *The Journal of Thoracic and Cardiovascular Surgery, 149*(3), 655–660. https://doi.org/10.1016/j.jtcvs.2014.06.032

Chapter 9
Confirmation Bias. Arthroscopy in the Treatment of Knee Osteoarthritis

The Problem

A placebo (Fig. 9.1) is a substance or procedure lacking specific therapeutic effect but used to simulate a real treatment. In the medical context, these are substances or procedures that do not have a specific pharmacological or pathophysiological action for treating a disease or condition. However, they are frequently used in clinical trials to compare the effects of an active treatment, with the aim of assessing whether these effects go beyond the psychological impact associated with receiving an intervention, also referred to as "treatment."

The word derives from the Latin verb "placere," meaning "to please," "to gratify," or "to delight," and corresponds to the first-person singular future tense of the verb, which would translate as "I will please" or "I will gratify." It was first used in a medical context in 1785, when it appeared in the second edition of George Motherby's New Medical Dictionary, where it was defined as a "useless medicine" or "trivial method" given to patients to calm them. Later, in 1811, *Hooper's Medical Dictionary* defined it more specifically as "any *medication prescribed more to please the patient than to be of benefit*" (Aronson, 1999).

The first documented use of a placebo in a formal controlled clinical trial is attributed to the American physician Austin Flint in 1863. At the time, Flint evaluated treatments for rheumatism, using highly diluted tincture of *quassia* (a plant) as an alternative (placebo) to the known treatment. Despite these early experiences, for many years the placebo was regarded merely as a curious phenomenon, and it was not until after the Second World War, with the work of Henry Beecher, that the placebo began to be recognized by the scientific and medical community as a factor to be considered and controlled in any research aiming to assess the true efficacy of a treatment. In the 1960s, the FDA and other drug regulatory agencies began to require more rigorous studies for the approval of new drugs, with control groups using placebos, thus establishing it as the current "*gold standard*" in the evaluation of any new treatment (Shapiro & Shapiro, 1997).

A. Sanabria and C. Betancourt, *Cognitive Biases in Surgical Practice*,
https://doi.org/10.1007/978-3-032-20377-9_9

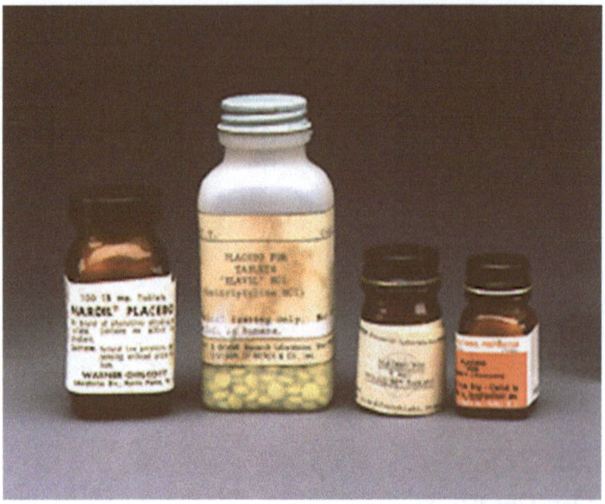

Fig. 9.1 Placebos (public domain). *Source* NIH, objects donated by Elaine and Arthur Shapiro—https://www.nlm.nih.gov/hmd/emotions/self.html

Currently, the use of placebos in pharmaceutical research to evaluate the efficacy of new drugs is a routine and mandatory practice. Despite this, surgery has remained largely outside this research methodology, based on the assumption that every surgical procedure is always beneficial and effective. This is explained by the fact that, in most cases, the indications for a surgical procedure and its potential benefits are sufficiently obvious to preclude debate, as is the case with appendectomy for acute appendicitis, splenectomy to remove a ruptured spleen following blunt abdominal trauma, or colectomy for the treatment of colon cancer.

The question that arises is whether this therapeutic certainty can be extrapolated to all existing surgical procedures. As has happened with many drugs, can a surgery not also act as a placebo? Along these lines, should we not consider evaluating every surgical procedure, especially those whose benefits are not so clear, against a placebo? Has this ever been done? Unfortunately, the answer is yes. And, to the concern of surgeons, surgical procedures have not fared well in these investigations. Among them, perhaps none is more enigmatic than arthroscopy for the treatment of knee osteoarthritis.

Knee osteoarthritis is a degenerative disease that affects the articular cartilage and the tissues surrounding the joint. It is one of the most common forms of arthritis and a major cause of disability. The condition results from the progressive deterioration of the articular cartilage, leading to pain, stiffness, inflammation, and limited mobility. Although this disease has been known for thousands of years, for many centuries it was confused with, named after, grouped with, and treated alongside other very different conditions such as rheumatism and gout. It was not until 1890 that Archibald Garrod, an English physician and pioneer in the study of inborn errors of metabolism, assigned the term in its current sense, noting that "osteoarthritis" was a disease "entirely distinct" from rheumatoid arthritis and gout (Dequeker Luyten, 2008). With a proper understanding of the disease, various treatment approaches emerged: lifestyle modifications and non-pharmacological therapies such as weight loss, heat and cold therapy, assistive devices, and physical therapy, along with the rational use of medications such as steroids and NSAIDs. However, in the absence of significant improvement, especially in the most severe cases, surgical alternatives were eventually introduced. Thus, the earliest attempts at arthroplasty aimed to provide a solution for the most advanced forms of the disease, characterized by severe joint stiffness or ankylosis. The original idea was to interpose a material between the bony surfaces to replace the articular cartilage, preventing fusion and thereby preserving some degree of joint function. Fat, skin, muscle, fascia, pig bladder, cellulose, and even gold sheets were used, but none yielded satisfactory or sustainable long-term results (Gkiatas et al., 2022). As understanding of the disease improved, surgical alternatives expanded and evolved into other procedures such as adhesiolysis, meniscectomies, osteophyte removal, joint lavage, and debridement. However, none of these attempts produced successful outcomes that would allow for their universal adoption. All of this changed with the advent of arthroscopy.

Popularized in the 1960s through the research and development of instruments and techniques by Dr. Masaki Watanabe in Japan, arthroscopy became one of the first minimally invasive surgical techniques to be developed, forever revolutionizing the way orthopedic surgeries are conceived and performed. The use of small incisions, improved visualization of structures, faster recovery, and reduced risk of complications quickly made it an alternative to conventional open procedures. Originally conceived and designed for the knee, arthroscopy also prompted the reconsideration and reevaluation of various procedures used to treat diseases of this joint, including osteoarthritis. Thus, traditional open techniques such as adhesiolysis, meniscectomies, osteophyte removal, and joint debridement, now performed arthroscopically, once again became central to the management of this condition.

By the 1990s, the general indications for arthroscopy in the management of knee osteoarthritis included its use for everything from diagnosis and defining the treatment plan to the application of specific therapies for concurrent problems (meniscal tears, ligament injuries, etc.), as well as the widespread use of debridement to "prolong the use" of the knee (Burks, 1990). In practice, it was used for any knee joint problem that resembled or could be osteoarthritis, despite the fact that the supporting evidence for such use was questionable (mainly case series reporting symptom improvement in variable percentages of patients), if not altogether lacking (Burks, 1990). Even more concerning, there was no pathophysiological basis to explain how these procedures could improve disease symptoms. Regardless of these concerns, its use only continued to expand in the following years. By 1996, it was estimated that in the United States alone, approximately 650,000 arthroscopies were performed annually for lavage and debridement due to knee osteoarthritis, at an approximate cost of $5000 per procedure (Owings & Kozak, 1998).

Amid this controversy, the Orthopedics Department at the Veterans Medical Center conducted a study that would resolve these uncertainties, becoming one of the most iconic studies in the history of medicine. They designed a randomized, placebo-controlled clinical trial, similar to those used in the pharmaceutical industry, to determine the efficacy of arthroscopic knee surgery as a method to improve osteoarthritis symptoms. Patients were divided into three groups: the first underwent arthroscopy with lavage, the second underwent arthroscopy with debridement, and the third received a sham or placebo surgery, in which they were given general anesthesia and superficial incisions identical to those in the first two groups, while the surgeon simulated performing the procedure using the same instruments and maneuvers as with the other patients. Postoperative management was the same for all groups, and even one patient in the placebo group developed a surgical site infection as a complication, which was managed with antibiotics. The results of the study would forever change the perception of arthroscopy in the treatment of knee osteoarthritis. To the surprise of most orthopedic surgeons, there were no differences in outcomes among the different groups. Arthroscopy was no better than sham surgery in relieving patients' symptoms (Moseley et al., 2002). Subsequently, several studies with similar designs found comparable results, and a Cochrane systematic review concluded that arthroscopy for the treatment of knee osteoarthritis offers no benefit over placebo (O'Connor et al., 2022). Currently, arthroscopy is not part of the standard management of knee osteoarthritis.

Beyond the revolutionary nature of the study and all its implications, it is difficult to understand why arthroscopy was used for the treatment of knee osteoarthritis for such a long time and in such a significant number of patients, when there were numerous unresolved questions regarding its effectiveness. There was no physiological or pathophysiological explanation for the supposed benefits of the treatment, and the scientific evidence that "supported" its use was questionable and circumstantial, derived almost entirely from case series and individual experiences. While the apparent improvement in patients can be attributed to the placebo effect of surgery, how can the behavior of physicians involved in recommending and performing these surgeries be explained? With so much information raising reasonable doubts about the utility of the procedure, why did arthroscopy become so popular? Weren't surgeons supposed to be the guarantors of the efficacy of the procedures they proposed? The answer likely lies in confirmation bias, the most prevalent of cognitive biases.

Definition

Confirmation bias is a cognitive process by which we tend to favor, search for, interpret, and remember information that confirms or supports our own beliefs and hypotheses, while disregarding, ignoring, or downplaying evidence that contradicts them, regardless of its quality. It is a common and highly influential psychological phenomenon that affects the way people perceive, process, remember, communicate, and even generate information. It acts as a kind of mental filter through which the brain only pays attention to, remembers, and values information that affirms or reinforces what is already considered true or, even more concerning, what one wishes to be true. Many consider it the most serious of all cognitive biases, as it allows erroneous ideas suggested by other biases to persist and take root in the mind.

In the example described, the physicians who planned and recommended arthroscopies believed in the benefits of the procedure for patients with knee osteoarthritis. When they later evaluated the outcomes, they identified patients who had indeed improved, and these "successful" cases, regardless of their number, actual cause, or the magnitude of the benefit, reinforced (confirmed) their belief in the procedure and its apparent effectiveness. From that point on, confirmation bias took over. Positive cases and any slight indication of improvement were amplified, remembered, and publicized; cases without improvement were attributed to other factors unrelated to the procedure (the patient did not follow instructions, was not an ideal candidate, not everything necessary was done, etc.) and were set aside, forgotten, or dismissed. In this way, despite evidence against the usefulness of the procedure, it persisted, with the well-known consequences of complications and increased costs.

History

The idea that human beings tend to obtain only information that validates their beliefs is not new. As early as ancient Greece and Rome, various thinkers and historians alluded to this tendency in their writings. During the Middle Ages, Francis Bacon, the English philosopher and writer who was a pioneer in the development of the scientific method, warned in his famous work *Novum Organum* about the human tendency to seek evidence that supports one's theories and to disregard evidence that contradicts them (Nickerson, 1998). However, it was not until the 1950s that this phenomenon attracted the attention of the scientific community, with the classic social psychology study by Hastorf and Cantril (Hastorf & Cantril, 1954). In this experiment, after attending a difficult and highly violent American football game between Dartmouth College and Princeton University, students from both universities were asked to record the infractions committed by each team. The results demonstrated that the same situation can be interpreted in diametrically opposed ways depending on each person's preferences and interests.

In 1960, Peter Wason conducted a series of experiments in which participants were asked to formulate and test hypotheses about theories, explaining the sequence of a series of numbers. His results showed that subjects tend to formulate and test hypotheses that support their beliefs, without considering those that could potentially disprove them (Wason, 1960). The bias would not receive its name until 1977, in the renowned work of Cliffor Mynatt, Michael Doherty, and Ryan Tweney from Bowling Green State University in Ohio. The authors created a kind of video game in which participants launched particles toward geometric figures with different shapes and levels of brightness. Some of these figures allowed the particles to pass through, while others repelled them. After completing the first two levels, where participants were free to shoot as many particles as they wished in any direction, they were asked to formulate an initial hypothesis about the rule governing the game regarding the ability of the particles to pass through the geometric figures. Once this hypothesis was defined, for the next ten levels they had to choose to play one of two alternate scenarios, depending on what they believed would be most useful for discovering the exact rule. These scenarios had been previously designed to represent situations that would allow for the confirmation, rejection, or testing of different hypotheses. After the game, participants were asked whether or not they maintained their initial hypothesis. The results were similar to those of Wason, with participants systematically seeking and observing information that supported their initial hypothesis, disregarding other possibilities, especially those that contradicted their assumptions (Mynatt et al., 1977). Multiple subsequent studies confirmed and expanded upon these initial findings, showing that there is no facet or area of human knowledge that escapes confirmation bias.

Impact

Confirmation bias is one of the most prevalent and powerful cognitive biases, affecting every facet of human nature and field of knowledge without exception. Its effects are numerous and varied. Among the most significant are:

At the Personal Level

1. **Poor and/or erroneous decision-making:** If one only looks for and pays attention to information that supports pre-existing or desired ideas, crucial data are ultimately ignored, which could otherwise lead to a more appropriate decision.
2. **Overconfidence with lack of learning and adaptation:** By giving importance only to information that confirms their own thoughts and beliefs, individuals become arrogant and self-satisfied. Feeling they are always "right," they process only information that suits them, failing to recognize that this reduces their ability to learn from mistakes and to adapt to new circumstances and information.
3. **Inability to empathize and reach agreements:** Being trapped in a biased view of reality, regarded as unique, plausible, and infallible, makes it impossible to understand and accept different perspectives that would allow for a broader view and understanding of the situation, and that would facilitate the creation of alliances and agreements beneficial to those involved.
4. **Lack of innovation:** By dismissing new ideas and proposals that are incompatible with previous thoughts and preferences, the same methods and tools continue to be used, which stifles creative capacity and leads to stagnation.

At the Collective Level

1. **Social and political polarization:** When individuals within a particular social group consume news or follow information sources that align exclusively with their own ideological and/or political views, "echo chambers" are created that merely reinforce preexisting positions. This limits exposure to differing ideas, leading to greater division and undermining the dialogue necessary for social growth.

2. **Flawed public policy design:** If politicians and other individuals responsible for shaping public policies only listen to and prioritize information and people that confirm their own views and agendas, they end up ignoring data that reveal unintended consequences or alternative perspectives, resulting in strategies that benefit only certain segments of the population.
3. **Delay in progress:** If, as a society, ideas or hypotheses that differ from those already held are dismissed and the same approaches are continually repeated, the ability to adapt to change may be lost. This leads to inactivity and to the lack of progress and growth that are essential for life in society.

Examples in Medical and Surgical Practice

The practice of medicine and surgery involves constant formulation and testing of hypotheses, from establishing the correct diagnosis for a patient to determining the best treatment strategy. Thus, confirmation bias can have a significant impact, with potentially dangerous consequences. Among the most important are:

1. **Increase in diagnostic and therapeutic mistakes:** When evaluating a patient, the physician forms an initial opinion about the patient's condition and the need for a specific treatment, based on this first assessment and previous similar experiences. This information represents a partial view of the patient's actual situation, which must be complemented with additional studies to confirm or rule out the initial impression. However, confirmation bias leads the physician to obtain and give greater weight to information that supports their hypothesis, while disregarding or undervaluing information that contradicts it. The consequences in terms of diagnostic errors and inappropriate treatment selection can be severe.
2. **Indication of unnecessary surgical procedures:** When focused on surgical solutions (as this is what the surgeon knows and prefers to do), the surgeon may underestimate or overlook conservative or less aggressive treatment options, which could be equally or more beneficial for the patient. For example, a surgeon who operates on all cases of acute cholecystitis without considering that some patients might benefit from antibiotics prior to surgery and a procedure only once the acute episode has resolved.
3. **Resistance to change treatment:** If the patient does not respond to treatment as initially expected, confirmation bias can hinder the reevaluation of the diagnosis or treatment plan, attributing the lack of improvement to the severity of the disease, the time required for the treatment to take effect, poor patient adherence, etc. Similarly, during a surgical procedure, it may cause the surgeon to persist with the same approach even when the findings clearly indicate a need for change. For example, a surgeon who continues with cancer resection despite clear evidence of unresectability.
4. **Selection of suboptimal techniques and/or surgical approaches:** All surgeons have surgical techniques, approaches, and ways of doing things with which they are more experienced, feel more comfortable, and have had success in the past,

leading them to consider these methods superior and more appropriate. These preferences may lead them to use such techniques in situations where they are not the most suitable, or to persist with them even when the circumstances suggest otherwise. For example, a vascular surgeon who always approaches the neck with longitudinal incisions, without recognizing that some patients would benefit from transverse incisions.
5. **Misinterpretation of scientific literature:** When reviewing studies or clinical practice guidelines, the physician may give more credibility and importance to those that support their preferred approach and be more skeptical of those that propose alternative methods or clearly contradict their own. For example, a surgeon who dismisses the option of active surveillance in papillary thyroid cancer because *"that does not fit my reality,"* without considering the evidence and real benefit of this management alternative.
6. **Delay in error correction with impaired learning and improvement:** If surgeons are unwilling to question their own beliefs and assumptions, the process of continuous improvement and the adoption of new and better practices are slowed and hindered.

How to Avoid Falling into Bias

1. **Acknowledge the existence of bias and be aware of your own vulnerability:** As with all cognitive biases, understanding their existence and scope is very important. However, in the case of confirmation bias, this first step is fundamental and indispensable, as it directly affects the way we process and accept new information.
2. **Cultivate intellectual humility:** Acknowledge the limits of your knowledge, understanding that no one knows everything and accepting that there are many things beyond your comprehension and expertise. Value truth above being right and prioritize the pursuit of reality, even if it means changing your opinions or admitting your mistakes.
3. **Question your own conclusions and engage in constant self-assessment:** Subject your own ideas to ongoing review, actively seeking flaws in your reasoning. Before forming any opinion or making any decision, ask yourself: How did I arrive at this conclusion? What evidence did I consider? And most importantly, what have I not considered? What am I overlooking? Did I truly consider the possibility that I might be wrong?
4. **Actively seek out diverse and opposing information to your viewpoints:** Conduct thorough research before forming a definitive opinion. Consult a wide range of sources representing the greatest possible variety of perspectives, paying particular attention to arguments and positions that contradict your own beliefs.
5. **Adopt critical and rational thinking:** Question the validity of all information you receive; do not settle for conclusions alone. Instead, inquire about the sources, how those conclusions were reached, and the validity of the methodology used. At the same time, acquire statistical and epidemiological tools that enable you to critically analyze scientific literature.

6. **Ask for and consider others' opinions:** Surround yourself with people who hold the widest possible range of viewpoints, actively seek out their perspectives, and listen without dismissing their opinions, especially those that challenge your own beliefs or hypotheses, aiming to find common ground. In work groups, encourage the participation of all members, regardless of their stance or role within the group, giving equal importance and consideration to everyone.
7. **Use the "pre-mortem" strategy:** Before making any major decision, imagine that you have already implemented it and it has failed spectacularly. Then, work backward and identify all the reasons why you might have failed. Once you have identified all these risks and blind spots, incorporate them into your decision-making process and assess whether you are still willing to proceed.

References

Aronson, J. (1999). Please, please me. *British Medical Journal*, 318(7185), 716. https://doi.org/10.1136/bmj.318.7185.716

Burks, R. T. (1990). Arthroscopy and degenerative arthritis of the knee: A review of the literature. *Arthroscopy, 6*(1), 43–47. https://doi.org/10.1016/0749-8063(90)90096-v

Dequeker, J., & Luyten, F. P. (2008). The history of osteoarthritis-osteoarthrosis. *Annals of the Rheumatic Diseases, 67*(1), 5–10. https://doi.org/10.1136/ard.2007.079764

Gkiatas, I., Sculco, T. P., & Sculco, P. K. (2022). The history of Total knee arthroplasty. In E. Hansen & K.-D. Kühn (Eds.), *Essentials of cemented knee arthroplasty* (pp. 3–14). Springer. https://doi.org/10.1007/978-3-662-63113-3_1

Hastorf, A. H., & Cantril, H. (1954). They saw a game: A case study. *Journal of Abnormal Psychology, 49*(1), 129–134. https://doi.org/10.1037/h0057880

Moseley, J. B., O'Malley, K., Petersen, N. J., Menke, T. J., Brody, B. A., Kuykendall, D. H., Hollingsworth, J. C., Ashton, C. M., & Wray, N. P. (2002). A controlled trial of arthroscopic surgery for osteoarthritis of the knee. *The New England Journal of Medicine, 347*(2), 81–88. https://doi.org/10.1056/NEJMoa013259

Mynatt, C. R., Doherty, M. E., & Tweney, R. D. (1977). *Confirmation bias in a simulated research environment: An experimental study of scientific inference.* Taylor & Francis. https://doi.org/10.1080/00335557743000053.

Nickerson, R. S. (1998). Confirmation bias: A ubiquitous phenomenon in many guises. *Review of General Psychology, 2*(2), 175–220. https://doi.org/10.1037/1089-2680.2.2.175

O'Connor, D., Johnston, R. V., Brignardello-Petersen, R., Poolman, R. W., Cyril, S., Vandvik, P. O., & Buchbinder, R. (2022). Arthroscopic surgery for degenerative knee disease (osteoarthritis including degenerative meniscal tears). *Cochrane Database of Systematic Reviews, 3*(3), CD014328. https://doi.org/10.1002/14651858.CD014328

Owings, M. F., & Kozak, L. J. (1998). Ambulatory and inpatient procedures in the United States, 1996. *Vital and Health Statistics, 13*(139), 1–119. https://www.ncbi.nlm.nih.gov/pubmed/9866429

Shapiro, A. K., & Shapiro, E. (1997). *The powerful placebo: From ancient priest to modern physician.* Johns Hopkins University Press.

Wason, P. C. (1960). On the failure to eliminate hypotheses in a conceptual task. *The Quarterly Journal of Experimental Psychology, 12*, 129–140. https://doi.org/10.1080/17470216008416717

Chapter 10
The Law of Triviality. The Keystone Project

The Problem

In 2004, a team of physicians from the Departments of Anesthesiology and Surgery at the Johns Hopkins University (JHU) School of Medicine, including Peter Pronovost, published a study (Berenholtz et al., 2004) demonstrating that the implementation of a multifaceted intervention, including both an educational activity for healthcare staff with a checklist establishing the minimum clinical conditions for vascular catheter insertion and the empowerment of nurses to ensure compliance, reduced the incidence of catheter-related bloodstream infections (CRBSI) in their intensive care unit (ICU) to nearly zero. After several previous unsuccessful attempts and interventions, this novel approach, which was not only simple but also cost-effective, established a new paradigm in strategies designed to reduce a condition affecting two million people and costing the US healthcare system over $4 billion annually. The information quickly spread to hospitals across the United States, giving rise to the *Keystone* project

The Keystone project (*Quality Keystone ICU project*) (Pronovost, 2008), conducted by JHU, the Michigan Health and Hospital Association (MHA), and the Agency for Healthcare Research and Quality (AHRQ), included 99 hospitals in an observational study to validate Pronovost's previous findings on CRBSI control in a more routine clinical setting. For its development, JHU requested a review by an independent research committee, which determined that, given the type of study (implementation of quality improvement strategies), informed consent was not required. In 2006, Pronovost and his team published their results in the *New England Journal of Medicine* (Pronovost et al., 2006), confirming a 66% reduction in infection rates.

However, on July 19, 2007, following an anonymous complaint, the *Office for Human Research Protections* (OHRP) reported that the study violated current research regulations by not considering participants as "human subjects," not seeking approval from an *Institutional Review Board* (IRB) at each participating institution, and not obtaining informed consent from each ICU patient or hospital staff member involved in the study. As a result, the OHRP ordered the suspension of all activities

A. Sanabria and C. Betancourt, *Cognitive Biases in Surgical Practice*,
https://doi.org/10.1007/978-3-032-20377-9_10

related to the *Keystone* project and its plans to expand the study to other states until the issue was resolved.

While the discussion between the regulatory body and JHU took place through correspondence, Atul Gawande, surgeon and columnist, who would later become director of the program that developed and implemented the World Health Organization's safe surgery checklists, wrote a review explaining the importance of these checklists (Gawande, 2007a), pointedly referencing Pronovost's example in the ICUs of Baltimore and Michigan.

Only 28 days later, on December 30, Gawande published a column in the New York Times (Gawande, 2007b), making the prohibition of the *Keystone* project public and criticizing it as "bizarre *and dangerous*." In his reflection, Gawande highlighted the differences between an experimental intervention (such as a drug) and an organizational modification aimed at improving quality of care, calling for a more sensible interpretation of the regulations, based on risks and benefits, to consider exceptions in cases like this and to apply research ethics regulations with the goal of protecting patients. The reactions were swift, and a growing number of criticisms appeared in newspapers and digital media (Gorski, 2008). Most expressed discomfort and disapproval of the decision, arguing that the OHRP had misinterpreted its own regulations and lost sight of its mission (Sabin, 2007).

On February 14, 2008, the OHRP re-examined the documents provided by JHU and Pronovost and acknowledged that, in fact, the study subjects did not fall under the regulatory definition of "*human subjects*" involved in research and, therefore, the invoked regulations were not applicable.

On March 27, 2008, representatives from the *Advisory Committee on Human Research Protections* and the *OHRP* met to discuss the various aspects of the controversy and its implications. Most arguments presented by participants in this meeting aimed to resolve a single issue: determining whether a study designed to improve the quality of care could be considered "*human subjects*" research. If these studies were classified as such, there would be a compelling need to obtain informed consent from each participant, thus fully justifying the suspension. If, on the other hand, they were not classified in this way, the suspension would not only have been unjust but would also have delayed the implementation of a life-saving procedure.

The meeting began with the participation of representatives from countless organizations interested in quality improvement projects and 63 internal and external experts from regulatory offices. The contributions, mostly consistent and redundant, presented arguments that clarified the particular nature of studies evaluating interventions focused on process improvement using strategies with demonstrated benefit (what were then called implementation studies, later grouped under the broader category of knowledge translation) and their distinction from those evaluating interventions focused on patients. At the end of the discussions, the director of the agency, in a brief statement, clarified that "*the case is closed and Johns Hopkins took actions to address the original problem, which related to decisions about exempt and nonexempt research activities. A current followup study now in progress no longer meets the criteria for human subject's research.*" On July 30, 2008, the OHRP finally authorized the reopening of project activities (Pritchard, 2008).

Currently, checklists are a mandatory part of medical and surgical practice. Their routine use saves lives by reducing the likelihood of catastrophic errors. The idea that at some point their implementation was limited by an irrelevant technicality now seems like a bad joke or a cruel prank. Yet it happened. The question that arises is: Why did it happen? How could a group of highly qualified individuals, genuinely committed to patient welfare, restrict their use? The answer probably lies in the Law of Triviality, one of the cognitive biases that most affects group dynamics.

Definition

Considered a key element of procrastination, the *law of triviality* (also known as Parkinson's law of triviality, or the "*bikeshedding effect*") is defined as the behavior in which people spend an excessive amount of resources (time) on minor and irrelevant decisions, and a lesser amount on crucial and important decisions.

When faced with a complex problem that requires multiple decisions, people must gather information for each of these choices. The greater the complexity of the decision, the more information and time are needed for analysis. However, in general, people tend to have more confidence, knowledge, and formed opinions about more mundane aspects (e.g., aesthetics) than about deeper issues (e.g., infrastructure). Thus, decisions that, due to their complexity, require more time tend to be postponed in favor of simpler decisions. This principle can be extrapolated to other types of resources besides time, such as mental and group effort, physical resources, money, and data. Although it occurs individually, its effect is much more noticeable in group activities (boards, meetings, consensus-building).

The most important contributing factors to the law of triviality are:

1. **The cognitive load required by the decision**: Cognitive load refers to the effort and demand on cognitive resources (attention, memory, etc.) that an individual must exert to perform a given task. People tend to delay or avoid these decisions due to the feeling of being overwhelmed by them (Ball et al., 2023; Gerhardt et al., 2016).
2. **The illusion of contribution**: The compelling need to feel useful and contribute to discussions on topics one is familiar with, but which do not entail significant responsibility or expertise and do not alter the overall outcome of the discussion (Silver et al., 2021).
3. **The Dunning-Kruger effect**: The mistaken tendency to overestimate one's knowledge or skills in a particular area (Dunning, 2011).

Nevertheless, it can also be seen as a conscious or unconscious strategy to avoid discussing difficult or challenging topics.

In the case of the Keystone Project, an unfounded complaint about a study with minimal risk and significant benefits was halted by the interpretation of a phrase by a regulatory committee that, according to the experts themselves, was irrelevant, inapplicable, and meaningless. Nevertheless, the situation escalated unexpectedly, with potentially catastrophic consequences for patient care. In the end, the discussion ended at the same point where it began and from which it should never have emerged, after the unnecessary expenditure of resources, time, and money.

History

Cyril Northcote Parkinson was an English writer and naval historian (1909–1993). While stationed in Singapore, Parkinson published the book that bears his name (Parkinson's Law) as a satire of bureaucracy (Parkinson, 1986).

Parkinson begins his chapter entitled "*High Finance or the Point of Vanishing Interest*" by introducing a scenario in which individuals form a finance committee tasked with making decisions on large budgets. These individuals are selected for this responsibility without technical knowledge or experience in managing large budgets being a requirement, as is often the case in many organizations. To this end, there is an organized agenda where the most important topics are placed at the beginning with the intention that they will be addressed and discussed in depth, while the less relevant topics, which are scheduled last, are dealt with more quickly.

Parkinson assumes that this arrangement is prone to error, affecting decision-making. First, people will make poor decisions, and second, the order of the agenda does not guarantee that the discussion will follow the intended pattern. He then describes a meeting in which a budget of £10,000,000 for the construction of a nuclear reactor is discussed. Several documents and technical analyses prepared by "*experts*" were sent in advance and are considered. The meeting includes people who do not know what a nuclear reactor is, others who do not know what it is for, and among those who do, few know how much it costs to build one. Only one committee member has extensive knowledge of the subject. When the discussion begins, the less informed members discuss the recommendations of the experts and suggest approval, while the most qualified member remains silent due to the complexity of explaining what a nuclear reactor is, what it is for, and because he believes the suggestions may be inadequate or incorrect. In the end, the topic is resolved in two minutes, and the meeting moves on to the next item, a bicycle shed with a budget of £350, where the discussion becomes more complex over issues such as the roofing material, size, etc. After 45 min, a budget of £300 is approved. Finally, the last item, concerning the provision of coffee for the welfare committee meetings, with a budget of £21, cannot be resolved after 90 min of discussion. From this example, the law is derived that explains how, in decision-making meetings, most effort is usually spent on irrelevant issues.

The topic was quickly adopted in administrative and management disciplines starting in the 1960s. In 1999, Poul-Henning Kamp, a Danish software engineer, revived this law, renaming it the "Bikeshedding *effect*," in a mailing list dedicated to discussing computer program design issues (https://bikeshed.org/).

Impact

At the Personal Level:

1. **Ineffective use of time and resources**. On an individual level, the law of triviality makes time use ineffective, as a huge amount is spent on decision-making with minimal effect on solving a given problem. It also leads to ineffective use of other resources (financial), allocating an exaggerated amount to less relevant activities.
2. **Inadequate focus**. This results in a departure from achieving the overall objectives of a given plan, as attention is focused on details that do not alter the outcome of an intervention.

At the Collective Level

1. **Insubstantial contributions**. In the field of surgery, the most significant impact is seen in multidisciplinary meetings for decision-making. In these meetings, all specialists involved in patient care come together along with a range of clinical, imaging, and laboratory data to clarify the diagnosis and determine a treatment plan. The dynamics of these meetings show that attendees are divided into "*active*" participants, who contribute opinions, and "*passive*" participants, who receive information from the meeting (Kane & Luz, 2011). It has also been shown that there is a correlation between participating and feeling that the meeting offers benefits to attendees, which can encourage participation even if the contributions are not particularly relevant. Furthermore, between 25 and 30% of attendees at these meetings feel that there was not enough time to discuss relevant clinical or treatment plan issues, as time was spent discussing imaging or pathology findings or irrelevant patient characteristics, such as whether the patient works in healthcare (*the "recommended syndrome"*) (Sanz Rubiales et al., 2002).
2. **Loss of the pursued objective**. Similarly, when evaluating the quality of multidisciplinary meetings (Ottevanger et al., 2013), concern for ensuring the technical conditions of the meeting (projection equipment, videoconferencing, etc.) is greater (>80%) than for more important aspects of decision-making (attendance of the specialists involved in the case (49%), advance provision of information for discussion (46%), and presence of administrative staff to follow up on the process (9%)).
3. **Changes in the order of priorities**. On the other hand, in meetings where all cases seen over a given period (weeks, months) must be presented without any specific selection criteria, the excessive number of cases affects the discussion of the more complex cases, due to the pressure to comply with the agenda (Hoinville et al., 2019).

Examples in Medical and Surgical Practice

There are countless examples of the effect of the law of triviality in medicine and surgery. Among the most frequent are:

1. **Unfocused Multidisciplinary Meetings**. Routine multidisciplinary meetings or "weekly case presentations" where no objective is defined and the discussion is driven by the novelty of diseases ("the rare case"), the difficulty of treatment ("the difficult case"), or the outcome of treatment ("the complication").
2. **Poorly Targeted Team Involvement**. Primary group meetings where "all those involved in the case" are invited, including personnel who have little to contribute to the specific decision at hand. For example, administrators in cases involving the choice between treatment alternatives, or clinicians without financial experience in budget meetings.
3. **Unstructured Morbidity and Mortality Conferences**. Morbidity and mortality conferences where the topics to be addressed have not been specified, allowing discussion of any aspect related to care. For example, a death due to an adverse event that ends up in a discussion about the department's budget, or preventable mortality that turns into an assessment of the residents' responsibilities.
4. **Leaderless and Unstructured Meetings**. Meetings without recognizable leadership, without time limits, and without the possibility for counterarguments or feedback. For example, informational meetings on planning led by a board representative without decision-making authority, or assemblies to discuss salary issues without a concrete action proposal.

How to Avoid Falling into Bias

1. **Establish an agenda or checklist**: To facilitate decision-making, using an agenda allows for defining the participants, the topic and objectives of the meeting, the expected time for each item, and the elements that support the discussion. It also prevents relevant topics from being overlooked.
2. **Focus the discussion and set priorities**: Surgical practice is often filled with meetings. Many of these are regular patient discussion sessions. In specific cases, it is necessary to reduce the number of topics or patients to be discussed (prioritize) to allow sufficient time for the discussion of a particular case.
3. **Separate decisions (into simple and complex):** If a meeting is expected to address several topics or patients, it is advisable for the organizer to analyze the complexity of each and estimate the time and effort required to resolve them (streamlining) (Walraven et al., 2022). Once this is determined, it is recommended to group less complex situations together and reserve those of greater difficulty for discussion in a longer time slot. For example, one meeting for critical cases and another for presenting service statistics.

4. **Designate a decision-maker**: The effectiveness of a meeting will depend on prior organization and proper leadership. At the end of the meeting, a conclusion is expected, whether or not there is consensus among participants. It should be clear from the outset who will be responsible for summarizing the information and deciding.
5. **Reduce group size**: Since a larger number of participants increases the need for each to contribute, whether their input is relevant to the discussion, limiting the number of participants to the minimum necessary ensures that the discussion does not become unnecessarily prolonged.
6. **Set boundaries**: When allocating resources (time, personnel, money, etc.), establishing minimum and maximum limits ensures that the discussion remains within these boundaries and prevents positions that are unrealistic or unattainable.
7. **Apply Tools That Enhance Meeting Quality**. Finally, there are multiple strategies aimed at improving the quality of decision-making meetings. The STEPS methodology has been evaluated in healthcare settings and provides a useful guide (https://edhub.ama-assn.org/steps-forward/module/2702508). Another example is the M&M Matrix proposed by Leo Gordon at Cedars-Sinai Hospital in Los Angeles, California, USA (Meyer, 1995).

References

Ball, S., Katz, B., Li, F., & Smith, A. (2023). The effect of cognitive load on economic decision-making: A replication attempt. *Journal of Economic Behavior & Organization, 210*, 226–242. https://doi.org/10.1016/j.jebo.2023.03.018

Berenholtz, S. M., Pronovost, P. J., Lipsett, P. A., Hobson, D., Earsing, K., Farley, J. E., Milanovich, S., Garrett-Mayer, E., Winters, B. D., Rubin, H. R., Dorman, T., & Perl, T. M. (2004). Eliminating catheter-related bloodstream infections in the intensive care unit. *Critical Care Medicine, 32*(10), 2014–2020. https://doi.org/10.1097/01.ccm.0000142399.70913.2f

Dunning, D. (2011). Chapter five—The Dunning–Kruger effect: on being unaware of one's own ignorance. In J. M. Olson & M. P. Zanna (Eds.), *Advances in experimental social psychology* (Vol. 44, pp. 247–296). Academic Press. https://doi.org/10.1016/B978-0-12-385522-0.00005-6

Gawande, A. (2007a). The checklist. *New Yorker*. https://www.newyorker.com/magazine/2007/12/10/the-checklist

Gawande, A. (2007b). A lifesaving checklist. *The New York Times*. https://www.nytimes.com/2007/12/30/opinion/30gawande.html

Gerhardt, H., Biele, G. P., Heekeren, H. R., & Uhlig, H. (2016). *Cognitive load increases risk aversion.*

Gorski, D. (2008, September 28). When human subjects protection stifles innovation, part II. *ScienceBlogs*. https://scienceblogs.com/insolence/2008/02/25/when-human-subjects-protection-stifles-innovation-2

Hoinville, L., Taylor, C., Zasada, M., Warner, R., Pottle, E., & Green, J. (2019). Improving the effectiveness of cancer multidisciplinary team meetings: Analysis of a national survey of MDT members' opinions about streamlining patient discussions. *BMJ Open Qual, 8*(2), Article e000631. https://doi.org/10.1136/bmjoq-2019-000631

Kane, B., & Luz, S. (2011). Information sharing at multidisciplinary medical team meetings. *Group Decision and Negotiation, 20*(4), 437–464. https://doi.org/10.1007/s10726-009-9175-9

Meyer, H. S. (1995). Gordon's guide to the surgical morbidity and mortality conference. *JAMA, 273*(1), 86–87. https://doi.org/10.1001/jama.1995.03520250102047

Ottevanger, N., Hilbink, M., Weenk, M., Janssen, R., Vrijmoeth, T., de Vries, A., & Hermens, R. (2013). Oncologic multidisciplinary team meetings: Evaluation of quality criteria. *Journal of Evaluation in Clinical Practice, 19*(6), 1035–1043. https://doi.org/10.1111/jep.12022

Pritchard, I. (2008). Indwelling Catheter QI Procedures: Letter, July 30, 2008. US Department of Health and Human Services. https://www.hhs.gov/ohrp/regulations-and-policy/guidance/july-30-2008-letter-to-dr-peter-provonost/index.html.

Parkinson, C. N. (1986). *Parkinson's law: Or the pursuit of progress.* Penguin. https://books.google.com.co/books?id=zcSqQwAACAAJ

Pronovost, P. (2008). Interventions to decrease catheter-related bloodstream infections in the ICU: The Keystone intensive care unit project. *American Journal of Infection Control, 36*(10), S171 e171–175. https://doi.org/10.1016/j.ajic.2008.10.008

Pronovost, P., Needham, D., Berenholtz, S., Sinopoli, D., Chu, H., Cosgrove, S., Sexton, B., Hyzy, R., Welsh, R., Roth, G., Bander, J., Kepros, J., & Goeschel, C. (2006). An intervention to decrease catheter-related bloodstream infections in the ICU. *New England Journal of Medicine, 355*(26), 2725–2732. https://doi.org/10.1056/NEJMoa061115

Sabin, J. (2007, September 28). Research ethics and quality improvement. *Health Care Organizational Ethics.*

Sanz Rubiales, A., del Valle Rivero, M. L., Flores Pérez, L. A., Hernansanz de la Calle, S., García Recio, C., & López-Lara Martín, F. (2002). [Recommended patient syndrome]. *An Med Interna, 19*(8), 430–433. (El síndrome del recomendado.)

Silver, I., Mellers, B. A., & Tetlock, P. E. (2021). Wise teamwork: Collective confidence calibration predicts the effectiveness of group discussion. *Journal of Experimental Social Psychology 96*, 104157. https://doi.org/10.1016/j.jesp.2021.104157

Walraven, J. E. W., van der Hel, O. L., van der Hoeven, J. J. M., Lemmens, V., Verhoeven, R. H. A., & Desar, I. M. E. (2022). Factors influencing the quality and functioning of oncological multidisciplinary team meetings: Results of a systematic review. *BMC Health Services Research, 22*(1), 829. https://doi.org/10.1186/s12913-022-08112-0

Chapter 11
Anchoring Bias. The Dysphonia of Kaiser Frederick III

The Problem

Friedrich Wilhelm Nikolaus Karl (Fig. 11.1), who would be crowned as Frederick III, Emperor of the German Empire in 1888, was a heavy pipe smoker. He had started smoking in adolescence, and by the age of 26 was a habitual smoker who spent his afternoons "*drinking coffee, smoking, and playing chess*" (Laurenson, 1995).

In January 1887, Frederick, then Crown Prince, began to experience dysphonia that worsened over the following days, prompting an evaluation by Karl Gerhardt, a Berlin internist, who diagnosed a vocal nodule and attempted to remove it orally on several occasions, without success. Despite multiple recommended treatments with mineral waters and changes of climate (available and advised at the time), the prince's dysphonia worsened. At that point, Ernst von Bergmann, a renowned surgeon and successor of Langenbeck in Berlin, attended to the prince, suggesting for the first time that the nobleman was suffering from laryngeal cancer, and proposed a partial laryngeal surgery, which at the time was rare and carried a high risk of complications (Minnigerode, 1986). Faced with this diagnosis, the royal household, encouraged by the recommendations of Otto Bismarck, decided to consult Morell Mackenzie, who at the time was a prominent English otolaryngologist (Fig. 11.2). In contrast to his German colleagues, Mackenzie considered that the condition was not a malignant tumor but rather an inflammatory disease for which surgery was not indicated. To corroborate his diagnosis, he performed several biopsies and involved Rudolph Virchow, (Hussein & Panning, 2018) a polymath and one of Germany's most important pathologists, regarded by his peers as the "*father of medicine.*" The reports from the initial biopsies concluded an inflammatory condition, which confirmed Mackenzie's view and led him to contraindicate surgery and maintain medical management.

Nevertheless, the heir's health continued to decline, and on several occasions, Mackenzie had to perform partial resections of the tumor to improve breathing. However, he continued to maintain his opinion that he was dealing with a benign

A. Sanabria and C. Betancourt, *Cognitive Biases in Surgical Practice*,
https://doi.org/10.1007/978-3-032-20377-9_11

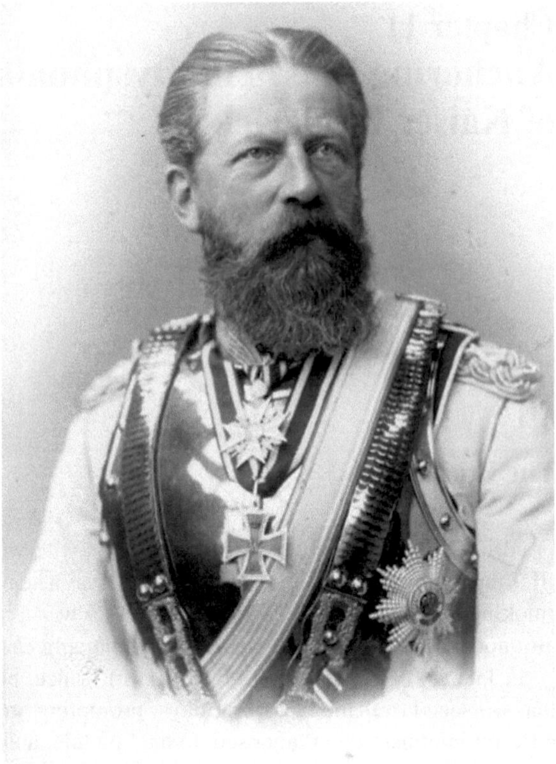

Fig. 11.1 Kaiser Frederick III. (Public domain image) (Reichard & Lindner. Portrait of Kaiser Friedrich III in uniform. Deutsches Bundesarchiv) https://commons.wikimedia.org/wiki/File:Bundesarchiv_Bild_146-2004-0099,_Kaiser_Friedrich_III.jpg

disease and that the procedures and topical treatments provided would aid recovery, even though this contradicted the recommendations of the German court physicians. These opposing views were communicated not only to Princess Victoria, the prince's wife, and the rest of the royal family, but also to the media in a biased manner. Over time, a dispute arose between the German physicians, who advocated for early surgery in the face of a disease that clinically exhibited all the typical findings of cancer (periodic recurrence of lesions despite resection, worsening airway obstruction, dysphonia, and general decline of the patient), and Mackenzie's opinion, who saw only signs of stability and spontaneous recovery and based his treatment on the biopsy results analyzed by Virchow. The controversies escalated, with mutual accusations and an evident denial by Mackenzie of the clinical evidence, leading to a new assessment by another pathologist, in this case Wilhelm Waldeyer, who confirmed malignancy. Despite the new data, the constant expulsion of tumor fragments, the suggestions of several colleagues familiar with the case, and the need for an urgent tracheostomy performed by a German surgeon, the public information never mentioned the diagnosis of cancer until the clinical situation became impossible to conceal. Clearly ill, Frederick was crowned Emperor after the death of his father, Kaiser Wilhelm I, and reigned for 99 days until his death from disease progression. The autopsy confirmed an extensive laryngeal tumor.

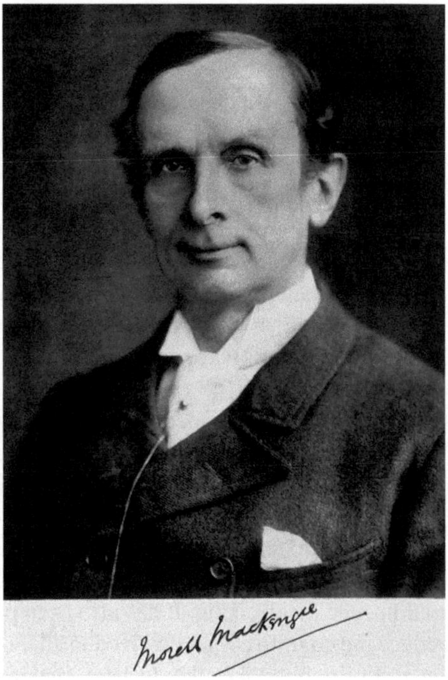

Fig. 11.2 Morell Mackenzie (Public domain image). https://wellcomeimages.org/indexplus/image/V0026772.html

After his death, the controversy continued until it could be confirmed that the clinical suspicions of the German physicians had always been well-founded and that, inexplicably, Mackenzie clung to his diagnosis of benignity and his proposal for conservative management (Laurenson & Levene, 1999). Amid the dispute, two extensive reports appeared, one German and one English, each defending its own position. Ultimately, faced with overwhelming evidence of a diagnostic error, Mackenzie was expelled from the English College of Surgeons for publishing confidential information that violated medical confidentiality and was repudiated by most of his English colleagues as well as by the new Emperor Wilhelm II.

Reading this story, it is impossible not to wonder how this could have happened. How could a renowned and highly qualified specialist repeatedly overlook the signs indicating that his initial diagnosis and subsequent treatment proposal were incorrect? How could he continue to defend it despite the patient's deterioration? Not even the patient's death was enough to change his mind. The fact that the patient was one of the most powerful and important people of the era only exacerbates these considerations. So, what happened? The answer likely lies in anchoring bias, one of the cognitive biases that most affect everyday life.

Definition

The anchoring effect or anchoring bias has been defined as a psychological phenomenon in which an individual's judgment or decisions are influenced by the first piece of information received on a topic (a point or anchor that is uncertain, irrelevant, and usually unjustified). This leads to an over or underestimation of new information, altering the ability to assess future events and causing the latest information to be disregarded or considered with less objectivity. It appears that the anchor persists for long periods in individuals (*longevity of anchoring*), and even in groups, its effect is similar to or even stronger than in individuals, specifically following the person who expresses the first opinion and sets the starting point.

Its existence can be explained by the *anchoring-as-adjustment theory*, which suggests that, once formed, the anchor always exists, with individuals using it as an internal reference point to adjust their decisions or responses, and that, despite attempts to correct for it, the adjustment is always insufficient. Another theory, called *selective accessibility*, suggests that people evaluate the anchor as a probable answer that requires external validation. When this evaluation occurs, it is not possible to detach from all the initial characteristics of the anchor, and, therefore, it continues to influence the decision. It has also been proposed that it may serve as a shortcut to reduce the cognitive load involved in analyzing a decision (*attitude change*). Having an anchor point makes the decision-making process and its cognitive demands less burdensome, so the information provided by the anchor is often accepted. It has also been suggested that the first information received on a subject is usually more easily remembered (*selective accessibility hypothesis*), so the anchor is established as soon as it is first observed.

Among the factors that modify anchoring (McElroy & Dowd, 2007) are mood (people in a positive mood are more resistant to the anchoring effect); experience and knowledge (experts in a field are somewhat more resistant, but not immune, to the effect of the anchor); personality traits (people with greater openness to experience are more susceptible); self-confidence (people with overconfidence are more independent in accepting external anchor points); and the way the anchor is presented (framing effect) (the use of round numbers gives an impression of greater magnitude) (Schindler et al., 2021).

In the case of Frederick III, the progression of the disease and multiple examinations suggested that the illness, initially considered benign, followed an atypical course for this diagnosis, with early recurrences and worsening of the patient's condition. However, a biopsy ruling out malignancy was used as justification to reinterpret these findings or even ignore them. The anchor was so strong that even new histological evidence, such as that provided by the second evaluation, was dismissed. It is difficult to know whether other political factors played a role in this process, but Mackenzie's obstinacy in clinging to his first impression and defending it to the end is evident. The disastrous consequences are already known.

History

Muzfer Sherif, Daniel Taub, and Carl Hovland, psychologists at Yale University (Sherif et al., 1958), published the first information related to anchoring bias in 1958, in a study evaluating the effect that a weight (anchor) had on the subjective assessment of the weight of other objects. They demonstrated that the anchor could shift the subjective assessment of weight in its direction, which they called the assimilation range. However, after a certain extreme value of the anchor, the opposite effect occurred, known as contrast.

Subsequently, Paul Slovic and Sarah Lichtenstein at the University of Oregon (Slovic & Lichtenstein, 1971), who had been working for several years on the psychology of decision-making, discussed differences related to the Bayesian approach to decisions, demonstrating the effect of initial values (a priori, anchor) on the determination of a posterior probability.

Finally, in 1974, Amos Tversky and Daniel Kahneman coined the term anchoring after conducting several experiments with anchors unrelated to the topic under discussion, which later became famous (such as estimating the number of African countries in the United Nations after spinning a wheel of fortune, and forward and backward calculation of a series of random numbers). They proposed the insufficient adjustment model as an explanation for the bias (Tversky & Kahneman, 1974).

Thomas Mussweiler and Fritz Strack of the University of Würzburg in Germany, in 1997, reanalyzed the original proposal of Kahneman and Tversky and proposed a new conceptual model to understand the psychological phenomenon underlying anchoring bias, which remains in use today (Strack & Mussweiler, 1997).

Impact

At the Personal Level:

1. **First Impressions as Persistent Reference Points**. Not only situations involving the setting of a numerical value are susceptible to anchoring bias. Opinions or decisions made within a group or community, such as a shareholders' meeting or a court, are also affected, where the first opinion expressed often shapes subsequent discussions (Bystranowski et al., 2021; de Wilde et al., 2018). Anchoring has also been demonstrated in interpersonal relationships, where a first impression of a person may persist unchanged, even if it is incorrect (DeCoster & Claypool, 2004).
2. **Initial Deadlines as Reference Points**. Another example of anchoring is the definition of timeframes for completing a task. The value initially set acts as the target, even if objective reasons later suggest that this first option was incorrect.
3. **Common Temporal and Social Reference Points**. Finally, anchors exist in all facets of life, for example, the age at which children can access certain benefits, the expected age of death, the time to be devoted to a particular task, or the

deadline set for making a personal change. Special dates throughout the year (Valentine's Day, birthdays, Black Friday) also serve as common anchors.

At the Collective Level:

1. **Decision Boundaries**. Traditionally, anchoring has been referenced in negotiation processes and its use in determining the starting point near a given value. In a negotiation, the first party to propose a starting point sets an anchor, while the second party, with their counteroffer, establishes a second anchor, between which the positions will shift. This subjectively determines the boundaries of the value of a particular object or decision (Caputo, 2013).
2. **External Reference Points in Negotiation Contexts**. Another area where anchoring is particularly strong relates to the setting of prices for goods or services. Once the anchor becomes popular, all proposals, whether from the same party or competitors, will remain close to this point. An analogous situation occurs when a third-party initiates with a value that must be discussed between two independent parties, such as in salary negotiations between employees and employers, where the state defines a starting point (Kristensen & Gärling, 2000).

The establishment of anchors is useful for navigating the complex world of decision-making. However, it has been shown that disproportionate or unrealistic anchors, which are difficult to achieve, can lead to dissatisfaction or incentivize unethical behaviors to reach these limits.

Examples in Medical and Surgical Practice

Several studies have shown that one of the most prevalent biases is anchoring bias (Ogdie et al., 2012). This is particularly ubiquitous during the diagnostic process and may account for 16–32% of complication cases (Antonacci et al., 2021).

There are several scenarios in which anchoring bias exerts its effect:

1. **Premature closure of the diagnostic process**, without conducting the appropriate diagnostic workup to confirm or rule out the initial hypothesis. For example, right iliac fossa abdominal pain in a woman of reproductive age that is quickly attributed to acute appendicitis, without considering other diagnoses.
2. **Establishing a starting point for the evaluation of subjective elements in medical practice, such as quality of life**: (Augestad et al., 2016). When measuring a highly subjective variable, if the assessment begins at a certain point, this value will influence the patient's responses. For example, an oncologic surgeon tells a patient prior to major cancer surgery that their quality of life is 100%, without considering that the disease may have already reduced it to 80%, thereby biasing all subsequent measurements.
3. **Defining therapeutic approaches based on hidden anchors**, which are taught and transmitted without considering the particularities of each situation. For

example, when considering a specific surgical treatment, an age over 65 may serve as a hidden anchor that prevents the use of major or complex surgical interventions or even leads to the denial of certain therapies.

4. **First impression**: When the surgeon interviews a patient, the first piece of information provided (symptom or sign) often serves as an anchor for the rest of the interview and the establishment of the diagnosis, even if later information contradicts or modifies the initial process (Ly et al., 2023). For example, in a patient presenting with a parotid mass associated with a prior infection, the first impression will be adenitis, even though other likely explanations include a primary tumor or nodal metastasis.
5. **Attributing all subsequent conditions to the primary disease**: When a patient is known to have a particular disease, all subsequent clinical changes are anchored to this condition, regardless of whether they correspond to the biological course of the disease. For example, a patient with a diagnosis of breast cancer who presents with unrelated conditions (cholelithiasis, diverticulitis, low back pain) will be investigated for metastatic disease (full-body imaging) and classified as having probable metastatic disease, even though pathophysiologically these conditions do not fall within the spectrum of breast cancer.
6. **Anchoring decisions in multidisciplinary meetings**: If, when a case is presented, the presenter establishes an initial line of thought, which can serve as an anchor to discuss only alternatives that are close to this first proposal. For example, in the discussion of a patient with abdominal trauma managed with an open abdomen and an initial proposal for reoperation, the discussion will focus on surgical approaches, complications, technical details, etc., while other non-surgical alternatives such as vacuum therapy are not discussed or considered.

How to Avoid Falling into Bias

1. **Awareness of the effect**: Being aware of the existence of bias, its theoretical explanations, and its consequences in decision-making can help protect against a greater impact on medical decisions.
2. **Identifying the presence of an anchor**: When deciding, reflecting on the arguments that led to the first impression or initial assessment can help mitigate the anchoring effect. Questions such as why this belief exists or who established a particular threshold can be useful.
3. **Challenging the anchor**: The Consider-the-Opposite (COS) strategy is one of the most useful tools. This involves compiling a list of reasons or evidence suggesting that the initial anchor is inappropriate, thereby questioning prior knowledge or beliefs (Mussweiler et al., 2000).
4. **Presenting multiple options**: When several anchors are offered instead of just one, the anchoring effect is reduced by establishing broader evaluation boundaries, allowing for a fairer comparison with other alternatives.

5. **Predetermining the anchor**: In group discussions that require decision-making, the prior establishment of a well-justified anchor helps protect against the potential anchoring effect intentionally or unintentionally set by other group members. This also applies to routine life activities such as when to retire, when to change jobs, etc.

While these strategies are useful in reducing the impact of anchoring bias (Webster et al., 2021) and there is empirical evidence supporting their use, the effectiveness of most of them is limited due to the ubiquity of the bias and its close relationship with others such as confirmation bias, availability bias, and overconfidence.

References

Antonacci, A. C., Dechario, S. P., Antonacci, C., Husk, G., Patel, V., Nicastro, J., Coppa, G., & Jarrett, M. (2021). Cognitive bias impact on management of postoperative complications, medical error, and standard of care. *Journal of Surgical Research, 258*, 47–53. https://doi.org/10.1016/j.jss.2020.08.040

Augestad, L. A., Stavem, K., Kristiansen, I. S., Samuelsen, C. H., & Rand-Hendriksen, K. (2016). Influenced from the start: Anchoring bias in time trade-off valuations. *Quality of Life Research, 25*(9), 2179–2191. https://doi.org/10.1007/s11136-016-1266-x

Bystranowski, et al. (2021). Anchoring effect in legal decision-making: A meta-analysis. *Law and Human Behavior, 45*, 1–23.

Caputo, A. (2013). A literature review of cognitive biases in negotiation processes. *International Journal of Conflict Management, 24*(4), 374–398. https://doi.org/10.1108/IJCMA-08-2012-0064

de Wilde, T. R. W., Ten Velden, F. S., & De Dreu, C. K. W. (2018). *The anchoring-bias in groups*. Elsevier Science. https://doi.org/10.1016/j.jesp.2018.02.001

DeCoster, J., & Claypool, H. M. (2004). A meta-analysis of priming effects on impression formation supporting a general model of informational biases. *Personality and Social Psychology Review, 8*(1), 2–27. https://doi.org/10.1207/s15327957pspr0801_1

Hussein, K., & Panning, B. (2018). Reconstruction of the examination of the laryngeal carcinoma of Emperor Frederick III by Rudolf Virchow. *Pathologe, 39*(2), 172–177. https://doi.org/10.1007/s00292-017-0392-8 (Rekonstruktion der Befundung des Larynxkarzinoms Kaiser Friedrichs III. durch Rudolf Virchow.)

Kristensen, H., & Gärling, T. (2000). Anchoring induced biases in consumer price negotiations. *Journal of Consumer Policy, 23*(4), 445–460. https://doi.org/10.1023/A:1007280722313

Laurenson, R. D. (1995). The emperor who smoked a pipe. *Journal of Laryngology and Otology, 109*(1), 1–4. https://doi.org/10.1017/s0022215100129111

Laurenson, R. D., & Levene, C. (1999). How the fatal illness of Frederick the Noble affected an Anglo-American friendship: Unpublished letters from Dr Morell Mackenzie to Dr Robert Myles. *Journal of Medical Biography, 7*(4), 234–242. https://doi.org/10.1177/096777209900700410

Ly, D. P., Shekelle, P. G., & Song, Z. (2023). Evidence for anchoring bias during physician decision-making. *JAMA Internal Medicine, 183*(8), 818–823. https://doi.org/10.1001/jamainternmed.2023.2366

McElroy, T., & Dowd, K. (2007). Susceptibility to anchoring effects: How openness-to-experience influences responses to anchoring cues. *Judgment and Decision Making, 2*(1), 48–53. https://doi.org/10.1017/S1930297500000279

Minnigerode, B. (1986). The disease of Emperor Frederick III. *The Laryngoscope, 96*(2), 200–203. https://doi.org/10.1288/00005537-198602000-00014

Mussweiler, T., Strack, F., & Pfeiffer, T. (2000). Overcoming the inevitable anchoring effect: Considering the opposite compensates for selective accessibility. *Personality and Social Psychology Bulletin, 26*(9), 1142–1150. https://doi.org/10.1177/01461672002611010

Ogdie, A. R., Reilly, J. B., Pang, W. G., Keddem, S., Barg, F. K., Von Feldt, J. M., & Myers, J. S. (2012). Seen through their eyes: Residents' reflections on the cognitive and contextual components of diagnostic errors in medicine. *Academic Medicine, 87*(10), 1361–1367. https://doi.org/10.1097/ACM.0b013e31826742c9

Schindler, S., Querengasser, J., Bruchmann, M., Bogemann, N. J., Moeck, R., & Straube, T. (2021). Bayes Factors show evidence against systematic relationships between the anchoring effect and the Big Five personality traits. *Science and Reports, 11*(1), 7021. https://doi.org/10.1038/s41598-021-86429-2

Sherif, M., Taub, D., & Hovland, C. I. (1958). Assimilation and contrast effects of anchoring stimuli on judgments. *Journal of Experimental Psychology, 55*(2), 150–155. https://doi.org/10.1037/h0048784

Slovic, P., & Lichtenstein, S. (1971). Comparison of Bayesian and regression approaches to the study of information processing in judgment. *Organizational Behavior and Human Performance, 6*(6), 649–744. https://doi.org/10.1016/0030-5073(71)90033-X

Strack, F., & Mussweiler, T. (1997). Explaining the enigmatic anchoring effect: Mechanisms of selective accessibility. *Journal of Personality and Social Psychology, 73*(3), 437–446. https://doi.org/10.1037/0022-3514.73.3.437

Tversky, A., & Kahneman, D. (1974). Judgment under uncertainty: Heuristics and biases. *Science, 185*(4157), 1124–1131. https://doi.org/10.1126/science.185.4157.1124

Webster, C. S., Taylor, S., & Weller, J. M. (2021). Cognitive biases in diagnosis and decision making during anaesthesia and intensive care. *BJA Education, 21*(11), 420–425. https://doi.org/10.1016/j.bjae.2021.07.004

Chapter 12
Loss Aversion Bias. Subspecialization in Vascular Surgery

The Problem

Since 1940, several general surgeons, members of the American College of Surgeons, developed the concept of *core surgery*, that is, *the fundamental surgical knowledge and training required for the care of patients undergoing surgical procedures on any part of the body*. This concept emerged in response to the perception that the integrity of general surgery, which had already seen the separation of cardiac surgery, head and neck surgery, pediatric surgery, plastic surgery, and ultimately vascular surgery in the 1930s and 1940s, was being threatened by increasing subspecialization (Jurkiewicz, 1989). These divisions resulted from the growing development of discipline-specific knowledge, the difficulty for general surgeons to keep up with scientific advances in each area, the need for specialized training in rare diseases, and the difference in clinical outcomes between surgeons dedicated to a particular field and those with a more generalist practice.

Other surgeons expressed concern about the "*drain*" of surgical cases from general surgery residents to future subspecialists, which would leave the former at a technical disadvantage. There was also apprehension about the tendency of certain subspecialty programs to recruit general surgery residents into their programs or to turn general surgery residents into a kind of servant under the control of subspecialists. Some even referred to subspecialists as "*Marauders on general surgery or raiders of the lost art*" (Wangensteen, 1985), while subspecialists viewed general surgeons as boundless hunters fighting over a fast-shrinking territory (Warren, 1974).

In 1946, nine general surgeons founded the Society of Vascular Surgery in San Francisco, California, with the aim of promoting the study and research of cardio-vascular conditions, standardizing diagnosis and treatment, unifying disease nomenclature, improving education, and advancing training (Yao, 2010). In 1962, Edwin J. Wylie established the first vascular surgery specialty program at the University of California, and in 1972, the two most important vascular societies (The Society for Vascular Surgery (SVS) and the North American Chapter of the International Society

A. Sanabria and C. Betancourt, *Cognitive Biases in Surgical Practice*,
https://doi.org/10.1007/978-3-032-20377-9_12

for Cardiovascular Surgery (NA-ISCVS)) proposed a formal body of knowledge and practice standards in vascular surgery, along with a request to create a Board of Vascular Surgery. Despite initial acceptance by the leading surgical organizations of the time (the American Surgical Association and the American Board of Surgery), formal approval was delayed for what vascular surgeons considered an excessively prolonged period, interpreted as an obstruction to the evolution of vascular surgery. These differences led the governing bodies to issue statements against the growing requests for certification of new surgical specialties, including oncologic surgery and trauma surgery, thereby blocking their approval as new certified specialties (Barnes, 1993). This tense situation was further exacerbated in 1974 by the proposal to create The American Journal of Vascular Surgery, which was seen as a financial affront that would reduce the subscriber base of general surgical journals and increase the number of "*mediocre*" articles (Warren, 1974).

The power battle continued for a decade until, in 1982, the American Board of Surgery accepted the creation of a special certification system for vascular surgeons. However, the disputes did not end there. The emergence of data showing that most general surgeons did not devote the majority of their practice to treating patients with vascular disease, and whose clinical outcomes were worse than those of surgeons with specific training in vascular surgery, combined with the trend toward an aging population and an increase in the incidence of chronic diseases, both risk factors for vascular diseases, underscored the need for recognition of vascular surgery as a specialty became more urgent. This request was made in 1997, accompanied by a document outlining the reasons why the existence of an American Board of Vascular Surgery was necessary. The subsequent response from the ABS, denying the request and stating that the proposal "w*as divisive, ill-timed, and not in the best interest of the larger surgical community, vascular surgery, graduate medical education, or the public*" (Stanley & Veith, 2016) fractured relationships and polarized opinions. As a result, two opposing factions formed within the American surgical community. Even in the first decade of the twenty-first century, the disputes remained bitter. The ABS continued to believe that recognizing the specialty would mean accepting the separation, compartmentalization, and fragmentation of general surgery and patient care, and therefore, an attempt to "*franchise*" surgical practice and a "*Balkanization*" of the parent discipline (Ritchie et al., 2000).

Simultaneously, the data revealed a different situation. In the United States, several studies evaluating the number of surgical procedures performed by general surgery residents in services where vascular surgeons were also being trained failed to demonstrate any significant detrimental effect on training (Perler & Zuidema, 1984). In Canada, vascular surgery became *de facto* an independent specialty from general surgery, with the recognition that this improved patient outcomes (Sidhu et al., 2003). It was even found that the creation of subspecialty programs attracted more interested applicants, thereby meeting the needs of both programs. Furthermore, the demonstration of an inverse correlation between a surgeon's procedural volume and mortality (the higher the number, the lower the mortality), particularly in major vascular procedures such as carotid endarterectomy, abdominal aortic aneurysm repair, and limb revascularization, strengthened the case for subspecialization. Finally, the reality showed a decreasing number of candidates applying to general surgery programs or remaining there without pursuing additional training (Grosfeld, 2002).

Today, after years of disputes, the ominous scenario of loss of autonomy in the training of general surgeons has not materialized, while the development of subspecialties has continued to progress and evolve, demonstrating that patient clinical outcomes continue to improve. The question that arises is why this dispute occurred. How could an initiative aimed at advancing and improving medical training, with clear and tangible benefits for patient care, be so strongly opposed? The answer likely lies in the loss aversion bias.

Definition

Loss aversion is the psychological tendency to perceive the loss of an object or opportunity as more painful (twice as much) than the equivalent gain. This triggers subsequent behavior focused on avoiding losses rather than obtaining gains (risk aversion) (Sokol-Hessner & Rutledge, 2019).

In this way, people opt for alternatives they perceive as safer and less risky in the short term, a phenomenon known as *myopic loss aversion* (*a bird in the hand is worth two in the bush*). In turn, when faced with alternatives with an elevated risk of loss, they prefer other options with less loss or even inaction, even if these are less effective (*better the devil you know than the devil you don't*).

Two theories have attempted to explain this bias:

1. As a cognitive mechanism, an implicit condition that causes individuals to act in this way systematically, even when faced with situations or conditions that are deteriorating (losses).
2. As modifications in information processing, where other factors unrelated to the cognitive decision-making process, such as emotions or excessive focus on loss, modify this decision.

The bias is less prominent in individuals in positions of power or with better financial conditions, as they can accept more dramatic losses without losing their status or have a greater ability to recover easily. There also seems to be less impact in highly cooperative societies, where individual loss is easily compensated by the community. Its impact also varies across different environments. Professional gamblers exhibit less loss aversion, while individuals with depression are more susceptible.

In the controversial dispute that arose during the emergence of vascular surgery as a specialty, in the face of a potential threat of reduced case numbers necessary for adequate surgical training or the perception of being limited in traditional areas of surgical practice (perceived loss), even without evidence that this effect would actually occur, general surgeons acted against the certification requests for vascular surgery. The sense of loss was so significant that these opponents of change were unable to clearly see the gains in patient outcomes and the improvement in training in areas where the number of cases performed is a guarantee of better results, as is the case with subspecialization. This led to persistent resistance to the formalization of the subspecialty, even in the face of current realities such as students' tendency to choose specific training, patients' demands for professionals with greater dedication and experience in a surgical field, and health services that continue to favor the creation of high-performance centers for complex diseases.

History

The topic has been discussed in psychological circles since the 1950s. Eugene Galanter of Columbia University, considered one of the fathers of cognitive psychology, and Patricia Pliner of the University of Toronto, had already evaluated in 1974 the value that subjects assigned to losses and gains without finding differences (Yechiam, 2019). In 1978, Peter Fischburg and Gary Kochenberger (Fishburn & Kochenberger, 1979), mathematicians at the University of Pennsylvania, reviewed a group of studies and were the first to design the well-known figure showing that the expected utility curve becomes steeper for losses and flatter for gains.

Based on these and other findings, in 1979, Daniel Kahneman and Amos Tversky (Kahneman & Tversky, 1979), psychologists, proposed prospect theory, whose main principle is that people do not make decisions according to the expected utility theory (which posits that individuals tend to maximize gains and minimize losses), but rather use a different decision-making mechanism that violates this economic theory. In a series of experiments, they demonstrated that participants assigned much greater utility to losses compared to equivalent gains. This theory added a perceptual and psychological dimension to the mathematical explanation of decision-making. Finally, in 1992, Tversky and Kahneman provided a solid theoretical structure for their proposal (Tversky & Kahneman, 2004).

The development of the concept of loss aversion was eventually extended to other areas of decision theory. However, today it is subject to various criticisms, and it is accepted that loss aversion acts preferentially when the decisions or bets under consideration are high stakes (greater absolute value in monetary terms), but its effect diminishes when dealing with lower values. Additionally, loss aversion is particularly strong when attention is focused on the loss (when there are only two options, win or lose), when the relative range of losses compared to gains is high (when the consequences of losing are greater than those of winning the same amount), and when it favors remaining inactive or at least does not incentivize action (if losing implies moving away from the current status quo) (Nagaya, 2023). It has even been suggested that people's predictions of the pain of a loss (hedonic loss) do not exactly match reality, and that, in the face of an actual loss, the emotional impact is much less than what was anticipated.

Impact

The impact of the loss aversion bias lies in its ability to prevent individuals from making better or more beneficial decisions, as the aversion to losing something is stronger.

At the Personal Level:

1. **Framing Effects on Purchasing Decisions**. Another common example of the impact of loss aversion is seen in the framing of a product's value. People are more likely to purchase a product if it is presented as a temporary discount (x% off for a few days) than if it is presented as a gain (buy three, pay for two), since in the first case, the time-limited discount is perceived as something that could be lost if not used. Similarly, in terms of services, people prefer to remain in a given low-quality service plan to avoid losing the benefits they have already acquired (bonuses, access to other services, gifts, etc.).
2. **Persistence in Unsatisfactory Long-Term Commitments**. In personal or work relationships, the bias acts to maintain long-standing but unsatisfactory or unproductive interactions (a marriage that has deteriorated over many years, a long-term job without career advancement), due to fear of losing them and the pain this might cause (sunk cost fallacy).

At the Collective Level:

1. **Risk Aversion and Investment Anchors**. The most common example occurs in financial markets and stock trading. Investors tend to hold on to stable or even clearly negative investments to avoid the pain of risking a loss with a new investment. They may also choose low-return but safer investments over higher-return options with a greater risk of loss. This tendency becomes particularly pronounced with increasing age.
2. **Risk Salience and Resistance to Change**. On the other hand, loss aversion reduces innovation because a successful project is not valued the same as a failed one, even if the overall benefits and losses are similar. A successful project may mean keeping one's job and a handshake, while a loss could mean dismissal. Thus, incentives to change the *status quo* decrease as the risks become more salient.
3. **Perceived Future Losses and Risk Protection**. Finally, all insurance companies are based on loss aversion. People perceive a future loss, even if unlikely, as more painful, and prefer to pay to avoid it rather than accept the possibility and suffer the loss.

Examples in Medical and Surgical Practice

Medicine, more than most professions, involves constant decision-making with the consequent evaluation and weighing of gains and losses (risks and benefits). In this sense, it is expected that the effects of the bias are multiple and diverse. Among the most important are:

1. **Maintenance of the Status Quo**: In which surgeons continue to do what they know and have mastered, despite the existence of better alternatives, to avoid losing comfort, control, or risking a poor outcome. For example, a surgeon who continues to perform open appendectomies on all patients, despite the clear benefits of the laparoscopic technique.
2. **Excessive Interventions**: To avoid the regret of a missed opportunity or the "*risk*" of a complication, which often exists only in the surgeon's mind. For example, a surgeon who prescribes prophylactic antibiotics for clean wounds to "*prevent*" a surgical site infection.
3. **Unnecessary and Counterproductive Comparisons**: In terms of economic revenue, general income indicators serve as a benchmark for comparison. If a physician falls below this indicator, they may feel they are at a loss and will adjust their behavior, schedules, and work methods to compensate for this perceived loss (Rizzo & Zeckhauser, 2003). This leads to performing more procedures per patient, shortening consultation times to see more patients, or prioritizing interventions with higher financial margins, among other behaviors.
4. **Unjustified Rejection**: Loss aversion is also observed in patients when the restriction of a highly valued, pleasurable, or useful item, such as high-calorie food, is perceived as more painful (a loss) than the future benefit gained in terms of obesity control, such as improved blood glucose levels or weight loss (a gain). This leads to a tendency to choose treatment options with no apparent losses (such as bariatric surgery), even if they carry higher risks. The same applies to other situations. A single episode of malfunction of a medical device is perceived as more painful compared to all the times it has worked perfectly, leading patients to avoid using it again despite its clear advantages. An unpleasant experience with someone (colleague, patient) is felt more acutely than all the positive moments shared with that person, resulting in the relationship being abandoned, and so on.
5. **Indiscriminate Use of New Technologies or Resources**: Another common strategy employed by the pharmaceutical and device industries is offering free trials of a particular product (a technology, a new laboratory test, a medication), which is then withdrawn after the evaluation period. This withdrawal is perceived as a loss, making physicians reluctant to stop using the product, even in the absence of clear benefits. This is combined with the continuous development of technology and its marginal improvements. The launch of a new product creates the impression that sticking with the old one constitutes a loss, prompting physicians to push for the acquisition of the new product. For example, a drug that offers only a negligible increase in survival but has just been released to the market.

6. **Distortion of Incentives**: There are payment models that leverage loss aversion to structure incentives for superior performance. In these cases, instead of awarding bonuses at the end of a period, the entire bonus is given at the beginning, with an evaluation conducted at the end. If the target is not met, part of the bonus is withdrawn. Since this is perceived as a loss of what was initially gained, physicians are more likely to meet the objectives.

How to Avoid Falling into Bias

1. **Recognize the existence of the bias:** Training or debiasing strategies using examples of how the bias operates can help reduce its future impact on decision-making (Hueber & Schwaiger, 2022).
2. **Consider all decisions related to the problem (portfolios) rather than isolated decisions (projects):** A comprehensive assessment of all decisions to be made can help mitigate the sense of loss in some of them (Sokol-Hessner et al., 2009).
3. **When initial failure is anticipated, focus on the outcome:** Since part of loss aversion is driven by the emotional impact on decisions, in cases where a loss is anticipated, extending the time horizon of the outcome can help mitigate the effect of this emotion. This involves exercises aimed at minimizing the cost or impact of losses (planning, creating reserves) or maximizing the gains from successes (awards, rewards).
4. **Let others decide for you:** Evidence shows that physicians tend to make less emotional and more rational choices than their patients in situations involving potential losses. Therefore, presenting the problem or decision to someone not involved in the issue reduces the effect of loss aversion. People are more impartial when they put themselves in someone else's shoes (Andersson et al., 2016).
5. **Make your responsibility for the decision public:** Having to publicly justify a decision leads to deeper analysis and more objective decision-making. The evaluation by external parties, which may be critical or unfavorable, can have reputational costs for the decision-maker, compelling them to guard against loss aversion (Vieider, 2009).
6. **Use objective tools to aid decision-making:** Some digital technologies (robo-advisors) can mitigate the effect of loss aversion, as they allow for a balanced assessment of alternatives, removed from emotional influences.

References

Andersson, O., Holm, H. J., Tyran, J.-R., & Wengström, E. (2016). Deciding for others reduces loss aversion. *Management Science, 62*(1), 29–36.

Barnes, R. W. (1993). Vascular surgery: The burr under the saddle. *Journal of Vascular Surgery, 17*(6), 1090–1094.

Fishburn, P. C., & Kochenberger, G. A. (1979). Two-piece Von Neumann-Morgenstern utility functions. *Decision Sciences, 10*(4), 503–518. https://doi.org/10.1111/j.1540-5915.1979.tb00043.x

Grosfeld, J. L. (2002). General surgery and fellowship training: Mutually beneficial or competing entities? *Surgery, 132*(3), 526–528. https://doi.org/10.1067/msy.2002.127696

Hueber, L., & Schwaiger, R. (2022). Debiasing through experience sampling: The case of myopic loss aversion. *Journal of Economic Behavior & Organization, 198*, 87–138. https://doi.org/10.1016/j.jebo.2022.03.026

Jurkiewicz, M. (1989). The college, general surgery, and fragmentation. *ACS Bulletin, 74*(11), 11–17.

Kahneman, D., & Tversky, A. (1979). Prospect theory: An analysis of decision under risk. *Econometrica, 47*(2), 263–291. https://doi.org/10.2307/1914185

Nagaya, K. (2023). Why and under what conditions does loss aversion emerge? *Japanese Psychological Research, 65*(4), 379–398. https://doi.org/10.1111/jpr.12385

Perler, B. A., & Zuidema, G. D. (1984). The effect of vascular fellowships on general surgical residency training. *Annals of Surgery, 200*(3), 247–254. https://doi.org/10.1097/00000658-198409000-00002

Ritchie, W. P., Jr., Rhodes, R. S., & Biester, T. W. (2000). Letters to the editor. *Annals of Surgery, 232*(1), 149–150.

Rizzo, J. A., & Zeckhauser, R. J. (2003). Reference incomes, loss aversion, and physician behavior. *The Review of Economics and Statistics, 85*(4), 909–922. http://www.jstor.org/stable/3211814

Sidhu, R. S., Ko, M., Rotstein, L., & Johnston, K. W. (2003). Vascular surgery training in general surgery residency programs: The Canadian experience. *Journal of Vascular Surgery, 38*(5), 1012–1017. https://doi.org/10.1016/s0741-5214(03)00611-6

Sokol-Hessner, P., Hsu, M., Curley, N. G., Delgado, M. R., Camerer, C. F., & Phelps, E. A. (2009). Thinking like a trader selectively reduces individuals' loss aversion. *Proceedings of the National Academy of Sciences, 106*(13), 5035–5040. https://doi.org/10.1073/pnas.0806761106

Sokol-Hessner, P., & Rutledge, R. B. (2019). The psychological and neural basis of loss aversion. *Current Directions in Psychological Science, 28*(1), 20–27. https://doi.org/10.1177/0963721418806510

Stanley, J. C., & Veith, F. J. (2016). The American board of vascular surgery and independence of the specialty. *Annals of Vascular Surgery, 37*, 4–240. https://doi.org/10.1016/j.avsg.2016.10.003

Tversky, A., & Kahneman, D. (2004). Advances in prospect theory: Cumulative representation of uncertainty. In *Preference, belief, and similarity: Selected writings by Amos Tversky* (pp. 673–702). Boston Review.

Vieider, F. M. (2009). The effect of accountability on loss aversion. *Acta Psychologica, 132*(1), 96–101. https://doi.org/10.1016/j.actpsy.2009.05.006

Wangensteen, S. L. (1985). Edgar J. Poth lecture. Changing prospects for the new surgical resident. *American Journal of Surgery, 150*(6), 650–654. https://doi.org/10.1016/0002-9610(85)90400-3

Warren, R. (1974). Editorial: Vascular surgery: Maturity or fragmentation? *Archives of Surgery, 109*(5), 603. https://doi.org/10.1001/archsurg.1974.01360050001001

Yao, J. S. (2010). Society for Vascular Surgery (SVS)-the beginning. *Journal of Vascular Surgery, 51*(3), 776–779. https://doi.org/10.1016/j.jvs.2009.12.029

Yechiam, E. (2019). Acceptable losses: The debatable origins of loss aversion. *Psychological Research Psychologische Forschung, 83*(7), 1327–2133. https://doi.org/10.1007/s00426-018-1013-8

Chapter 13
The Halo Effect. The Shah of Iran's Cancer

The Problem

On January 16, 1979, Mohammad Reza Pahlevi, until then the Shah of Iran and the last representative of a monarchy that had lasted more than 2,500 years, left his country after 38 years in power. Piloting the plane himself, accompanied only by his royal guard and a few journalists, he headed to Egypt on a trip officially described as vacation. The reality, however, was quite different. His own prime minister, Shapour Bakhtiar, had asked him to step down and leave the country in an attempt to quell the severe protests and strikes called by the Islamic Revolution of the ayatollahs, which had rendered Iran completely ungovernable. It had all begun fifteen years earlier, in 1963, when, following a failed coup attempt, the Shah launched a sweeping program of political, economic, and social reforms known as the "*White Revolution.*" Land and property redistribution, industrialization, women's suffrage and the removal of dress restrictions, literacy campaigns, and military modernization, among other initiatives, formed the pillars of these reforms. Although they had their supporters, the ayatollahs (priests and experts in Islamic doctrine) opposed them, viewing them as a form of "*Westernization*" and abandonment of the "*good customs*" that were a fundamental component of Islamic society. Thus, Ayatollah Khomeini led a series of protests that left more than 20,000 injured and culminated in his exile in 1964. Despite the apparent calm that followed, the seeds of discontent had been sown in Iranian society and continued to be nurtured by the ayatollahs from their religious centers and through the distribution of cassette tapes sent by Khomeini. The harsh repression, social control, and imprisonments with which the Shah tried to address the situation, combined with a severe economic crisis caused by government corruption, only increased social instability. In early 1978, the ayatollahs called for protests and strikes across the country in what they called the "*Islamic Revolution,*" which would ultimately lead to the Shah's departure (Keddie & Richard, 2003).

Beyond the political, economic, and social turmoil caused by the loss of power, the Shah faced even more serious personal concerns. In 1974, two French hematologists

A. Sanabria and C. Betancourt, *Cognitive Biases in Surgical Practice*,
https://doi.org/10.1007/978-3-032-20377-9_13

were brought to Tehran, ostensibly to evaluate an Iranian minister, but on the night of their arrival they discovered that their real patient was the Shah. Over 50 years old and apparently healthy, the Shah had been complaining for several months of a mass sensation under his left lower ribs, along with some palpable cervical lymph nodes. The French doctors had been brought in on the condition that there would be no record of the illness, nor any imaging studies or biopsies. After a clinical evaluation and some laboratory tests, the hematologists diagnosed the Shah with an indolent form of non-Hodgkin lymphoma and decided to begin treatment (Khoshnood & Khoshnood, 2016). Thus, as he left his country, the deposed monarch was also burdened with a serious health problem.

After visiting several countries in search of asylum and protection, the Shah settled in Cuernavaca, Mexico. Several months later, he began to develop jaundice, fever, and weight loss. Although malaria was initially suspected, he was eventually diagnosed with gallstones and choledocholithiasis requiring surgical treatment. For this procedure, he was taken to the United States on October 22, 1979. The operation was successfully performed at New York Hospital by Dr. Bjorn Thorbjarnarson, a distinguished disciple of the renowned hepatobiliary surgeon Frank Glenn. Although the surgery and postoperative course were uneventful, splenomegaly was noted during the operation. This, together with the recurrence of cervical lymphadenopathy, made it clear that the lymphoma had returned. Evaluated by a team of oncologists at Memorial Sloan-Kettering Cancer Center, he was prescribed radiotherapy, after which the lymph nodes disappeared, but the splenomegaly persisted and it became increasingly apparent that surgery would be necessary. However, on the other side of the world, an event occurred that prevented the Shah's treatment from continuing in the United States.

On November 4, 1979, a mob of revolutionary agitators in Teheran, under the protection and assistance of the new government, stormed the American embassy, taking hostage the 66 people inside. They demanded the immediate extradition of the Shah, threatening to kill one hostage every 24 h if their demands were not met. Faced with this situation, the U.S. government decided to arrange for the Shah's departure, first to Mexico and then to Egypt, where it became clear that splenic surgery could no longer be postponed. After discussions among the Shah's medical team and Egyptian and American authorities, it was decided that the procedure should not be performed by just any surgeon, but by the best possible surgeon. With the ability to choose virtually anyone in the world, the selection was none other than the world-renowned Dr. Michael DeBakey (Asz et al., 2005).

At this point, DeBakey was without question the most famous and acclaimed surgeon in the world. A pioneer in cardiovascular surgery, he had developed a series of innovations in surgical technique and instrumentation that had enabled previously unimaginable advances in this field. In particular, his new surgical techniques for myocardial revascularization and the management of aortic dissection had made possible to treat these previously almost invariably fatal conditions. Surgeons from around the world traveled to Houston, where he served as chief of surgery at Baylor University, to observe and learn from his work. His precision and elegance in the operating room, along with his extraordinary results, had earned him the nickname "*The*

Master," by which he was known worldwide. His fame extended beyond the medical community, with his patients including heads of state, celebrities, and athletes from around the globe. Among them were King Edward VIII of England, U.S. Presidents John F. Kennedy and Richard Nixon, King Hussein of Jordan, magnate Aristotle Onassis, and German actress Marlene Dietrich, to name just a few of the most prominent. (Eads & Ikonomidis, 2014) Thus, when the deposed Shah of Iran required a surgeon for a splenectomy, the choice was quite obvious. The fact that DeBakey was a cardiovascular surgeon did not seem to be a concern.

On March 28, 1980, at the Maadi Military Hospital in Cairo, accompanied by his closest assistants and the head of the surgical department, Dr. Nour, DeBakey performed the Shah's splenectomy. Despite some details that became known later (during ligation of the splenic hilum, Nour warned DeBakey that the tail of the pancreas was being transected but was ignored; his suggestion to place a drain was also not heeded), the surgery was reported as an absolute success. DeBakey himself, at a press conference, announced that the Shah's health was "*very satisfactory*" and that he could "*live for many years*" (Ibrahim, 1980). The spleen weighed about 2 kg, and pathology reported Waldenstrom's macroglobulinemia, a rare and indolent form of lymphoma. Unfortunately, microscopic examination also found pancreatic tissue in the splenic hilum. On the third postoperative day, the Shah developed left shoulder pain and fever, which was initially managed expectantly due to the absence of abdominal symptoms or signs and his generally good condition. As symptoms persisted, pneumonia was diagnosed and antibiotic treatment was started. The Shah's condition gradually deteriorated, and after three months of intermittent antibiotic therapy, multiple evaluations by various specialists, and a bronchoscopy negative for infection, a left subphrenic abscess was diagnosed. The Shah underwent another operation for drainage on June 27, 1980, and although he experienced brief improvement, he collapsed three weeks later, victim of massive intra-abdominal hemorrhage related to a pancreatic fistula. After three operations, the Shah died on July 27, 1980. He was 60 years old (van de Laar, 2024).

Beyond the complication inherent to any surgical practice, questions arise regarding the process that led to DeBakey being considered the most suitable person to perform the splenectomy. Although he had been exposed to abdominal surgery during his training, at the time of the call, DeBakey had spent more than fifteen years exclusively dedicated to cardiovascular surgery. Despite his skill as a surgeon, such a long absence from abdominal surgery could not be overlooked, especially in a complex case like the Shah's. If there is one important thing in surgery, it's the repetition and constant practice of surgical procedures.

So, why was "*The Master*" chosen? The Shah was an immensely wealthy man with highly influential friends, so lack of connections or financial constraints do not seem to have been significant factors. Although the monarch was not an expert in the field, his medical team included Iranian, American, French, and Egyptian specialists from various disciplines, several of whom were surgeons who clearly understood the competencies of the different surgical specialties, ruling out ignorance. Being in exile and under the protection of the U.S. and Egyptian governments, it is almost impossible to think that the Shah was forced to choose DeBakey. On the other hand, six months earlier, the Shah had undergone successful surgery by a hepatobiliary surgeon, so a previous bad experience was not the case. In fact, given this precedent and considering that Dr. Thorbjarnarson was indeed an expert in the field and already knew the Shah, the real question is why he was not chosen. So, why did a team of highly qualified individuals, with countless options at their disposal, end up choosing someone who, despite all his credentials, fame, and achievements, was clearly not the best option for this surgery? The answer probably lies in one of the cognitive biases used daily in the world of advertising, such as the halo effect.

Definition

The halo effect is defined as the biased cognitive process by which skills, abilities, or attributes of a person or particular situation are inferred based on what is known about that person or situation, usually a single striking aspect or characteristic. It is difficult for the human brain to independently judge each characteristic of a person or situation; therefore, we tend to evaluate them collectively, creating a consistent and coherent image. As with all cognitive biases, a difficult question is replaced by an easier one. In the specific case of this bias, the difficult question of how qualified a person is and what they know about a particular subject is replaced by what I know about this person. If the person excels at what they do, is pleasant, attractive, etc., it is assumed that the person is qualified, trustworthy, and even an expert in the area they are commenting on. Conversely (some have referred to this as the *Horn effect*), if what I know about a person is negative, because they have made mistakes in previous statements, are unpleasant, or even unattractive, it is then inferred that they are not trustworthy, not qualified, and must not know anything about the subject at hand. The same occurs when judging other situations. The difficult question, for example: how concerned I should be about this situation, is replaced by the easier one, what do I know about the situation. Favorable answers will lead to considering the situation as not very concerning, and unfavorable answers will lead to considering it as very concerning. The halo effect generates an unconscious, entirely subjective, and unreliable evaluation process of a person or situation, since the characteristics of a particular aspect of a person or situation do not define the characteristics of other aspects. In the vast majority of cases, they are not even related.

In the specific case of the selection of DeBakey by the Shah's medical team, the difficult question of who was the most qualified surgeon *to perform a splenectomy* was replaced by the easier question of who is the most qualified surgeon. When DeBakey's name came up, with all his attributes, fame, and recognition, the halo effect led to the assumption that, just as he was brilliant in cardiovascular surgery, he must also be so in performing a splenectomy. The consequences are well known.

History

The halo effect was first described in 1920 by Edward L. Thorndike while conducting studies on psychological evaluations of military personnel (Thorndike, 1920). In the study, officers were asked to evaluate a series of qualities of their subordinates. Upon analyzing the data, Thorndike observed that the way specific characteristics were evaluated was directly related to how the rest of the other characteristics were assessed. Soldiers who received negative ratings in one area also received negative ratings in other evaluated characteristics. The same occurred with those who received positive ratings. Multiple studies have confirmed these initial findings and expanded our understanding of bias. Of particular importance is the work of Solomon Asch, who showed that in the absence of other information, we tend to judge people by their physical attractiveness (Asch, 1946), and that of Nisbett and Wilson, who demonstrated that we are completely unaware of how the halo effect influences our evaluations (Nisbett & Wilson, 1977).

Impact

The halo effect affects the way people are evaluated in daily interactions and the situations we face. Among the most important are:

At the Personal Level:

1. **Estimation of attributes or abilities:** When it is necessary to determine an unknown aspect of a person, instead of gathering information that would allow for an appropriate conclusion, judgment is based on other aspects of the person that are already known. Thus, for example, if a person is very pleasant, they will also be considered responsible, even though both sides may be entirely unrelated.
2. **Evaluation of situations:** When facing unknown situations, instead of conducting relevant research, we tend to make judgments based on the little we know about them, which, in many cases, may be completely irrelevant data for the evaluation. For example, when deciding whether to invest in a particular product, the decision is made based on whether the product appears attractive or not, which is irrelevant when determining the product's success.
3. **The problem of first impressions:** Much has been said and written about the importance of first impressions. In light of our understanding of the halo effect, we should reconsider this belief. When meeting someone for the first time, it is impossible to determine if the person is responsible, trustworthy, capable, conciliatory, etc. At best, one can tell if the person is pleasant and/or attractive. However, from this limited observation, the halo effect creates in the mind an image of the person consistent with this first impression. Thus, for example, if the person is pleasant, they will be considered trustworthy. As Solomon Asch

demonstrated in his work, if the person is unattractive, they will be considered less qualified, distant, untrustworthy, etc.

At the Collective Level:

1. **Product evaluation:** The halo effect is used in advertising campaigns to ensure that the public evaluates new product launches positively. When new products from well-known brands are introduced, instead of judging the product from scratch and gathering objective information about it, an automatic association is made between brand recognition and product quality, aspects that are not necessarily related.
2. **Acceptance of messages and social recognition:** Attractive and pleasant individuals have greater ease in accessing leadership positions and in having their messages accepted. The collective and/or political implications of this are concerning. Due to the Halo effect, it is very likely that we end up accepting and considering as true the messages of those leaders who appear likable, friendly, and good-looking, qualities that clearly have no relation to the individual's suitability for a given position. Similarly, we may end up dismissing the most qualified person simply because they are not cordial or humorous.

Examples in Medical and Surgical Practice

As a profession that is constantly exposed to new people, problems, and situations, the halo effect extends its influence on every facet of a surgeon's practice. Among the most important are:

1. **Acceptance or questioning of difficult or controversial diagnostic situations** based on the expertise of the person making the diagnosis in their field. For example, if a renowned radiation oncologist establishes a diagnosis of sclerosing cholangitis, it is more likely to be accepted compared to if it comes from a newly graduated general practitioner.
2. **Proposing more favorable diagnoses** depending on how pleasant or likable the patient seems. In situations of doubt or in the absence of solid evidence, there is a tendency to propose more favorable diagnoses for patients who appear cordial, sociable, etc.
3. **Prescription of medications based on the laboratory or commercial brand that produces them**, especially in situations where the evidence is unclear. For example, the slogan "*If it's Bayer, it's good*," introduced by the pharmaceutical company during the 1980s in response to the uncertainty at the time regarding the widespread use of antiplatelet agents for the prevention of cardiovascular events.
4. **Widespread use of new technologies** at the suggestion of "*leading*" companies in the market. For example, if a medical device is produced in Japan, it is assumed to have the same quality as other Japanese technologies, such as automobiles.

5. **Adoption of new behaviors or procedures** after being presented by world-renowned figures. For example, starting to recommend a certain orthopedic treatment after learning about the "*fabulous*" experience and its subsequent endorsement by a famous soccer player.
6. **Greater recommendation of curative treatments in borderline situations** with uncertain chances of success, depending on our opinion of the patient. Faced with the same scenario, there is a tendency to offer more curative treatments to patients about whom there are positive perceptions or opinions, considering them to have a greater chance of "*cure*."
7. **Tendency to accept or dismiss the opinions of others based on their "*expertise*"** in meetings where patient management decisions are made. It is more likely to accept and follow the opinion of the head of the hematology department than that of a second-year surgery resident.

How to Avoid Falling into This Bias

Eradicating the halo effect is practically impossible, as evaluating and categorizing each particular facet of every person or situation separately would be extremely exhausting for the brain. However, there are a series of strategies that can be used to limit its impact, especially in critical situations. Among these are:

1. **Learn to categorize and evaluate each person or situation solely based on what is known, prioritizing neutrality:** As with all cognitive biases, the first step is to be aware of its existence and the impact it has on mental processes. Thus, in the case of the halo effect, one must begin by recognizing that only certain aspects of the people around us or the situations we face are known, and that from these, we cannot assume what the other aspects are like, acknowledging that inconsistencies exist. In this way, someone may be an expert in a particular field and at the same time completely ignorant in others, just as someone may be very pleasant and at the same time completely irresponsible. In this sense, it is essential to categorize people only based on what is known with certainty, leaving what is unknown in complete neutrality.
2. **Practice skepticism:** As tedious as it may be, in every new situation that must be faced, one should start from a point of total skepticism, while building a view of people and situations based on tangible and objective facts that allow for correct evaluations.
3. **Use objective, standardized, and, if possible, blinded tests or assessment tools:** When evaluating new medications, technologies, procedures, and even scientific information, use standardized tools focused on objective measures of performance or function that allow for the exclusion of subjective aspects that may be influenced by the Halo effect. Likewise, as far as possible, try to remain blind to the manufacturer, company, brand, author, or medical center where the product under consideration came from.

4. **Involve multiple observers:** For those cases where the previous recommendation cannot be applied, such as evaluating people, where interaction is essential, instead of relying on an individual perspective, let the final opinion rest with a group of people, ideally each with different backgrounds, training, perspectives, interests, etc. In this way, the outcome of the final evaluation will be more objective, as it is unlikely that the Halo effect will influence all participants equally.
5. **Be wary of first impressions:** The Halo effect leads us to make assumptions about a person based on a first encounter, which is too limited for such inferences. While ideally nothing should be assumed after a first impression, the way the brain works makes this virtually impossible. Therefore, recognize the limitations of first impressions, understanding that no matter how pleasant or well presented a person may be, anything beyond that is merely a supposition and, as such, is likely to be incorrect.

References

Asch, S. E. (1946). *Forming impressions of personality.* https://doi.org/10.1037/h0055756

Asz, S., Fernández, S., & Cervantes, C. (2005). Mexico and the political crisis due to the illness of the Shah of Iran. *Cir Gen, 27*(1), 86–89.

Eads, D., & Ikonomidis, J. S. (2014). Historical perspectives of The American Association for Thoracic Surgery: Michael E. DeBakey (1908–2008). *The Journal of Thoracic and Cardiovascular Surgery, 147*(4), 1123–1127. https://doi.org/10.1016/j.jtcvs.2013.12.029

Ibrahim, Y. (1980, March 30). Surgery to remove Shah's Spleen is called successful; Spleen had ceased to function. *The New York Times.* https://www.nytimes.com/1980/03/30/archives/surgery-to-remove-shahs-spleen-is-called-successful-spleen-had.html

Keddie, N. R., & Richard, Y. (2003). *Modern Iran: Roots and results of revolution.* Yale University Press. https://books.google.com.co/books?id=DgHhdALiAxIC

Khoshnood, A., & Khoshnood, A. (2016). The death of an emperor—Mohammad Reza Shah Pahlavi and his political cancer. *Alexandria Journal of Medicine, 52*(3), 201–208. https://doi.org/10.1016/j.ajme.2015.11.002

Nisbett, R. E., & Wilson, T. D. (1977). Telling more than we can know: Verbal reports on mental processes. *Psychological Review, 84*(3), 231–259. https://doi.org/10.1037/0033-295X.84.3.231

Thorndike, E. L. (1920). A constant error in psychological ratings. *Journal of Applied Psychology, 4*(1), 25–29. https://doi.org/10.1037/h0071663

van de Laar, A. (2024). *Under the knife: A history of surgery in 28 remarkable operations.* St. Martin's Press. https://books.google.com.co/books?id=pJVJDwAAQBAJ

Chapter 14
Overconfidence Bias. Benjamin Rush and the Yellow Fever Epidemic of 1793

The Problem

By 1793, Philadelphia was the largest city in the United States. Its prime location on the Delaware River facilitated trade with Europe and the Caribbean, making it the nation's largest and busiest port. This had established it as the main financial center, home to the first bank and the first stock exchange. Moreover, the events that took place in the city during and after the War of Independence (the Declaration of Independence was signed in Philadelphia in 1776 and the United States Constitution in 1787) had given it unparalleled political and historical significance, making it the temporary capital of the nascent United States and the seat of the main federal institutions while the new permanent capital, Washington DC, was under construction. By the late eighteenth century, it was also the place of residence and work for all the leading figures of the United States. George Washington, Benjamin Franklin, Thomas Jefferson, Alexander Hamilton, and many others lived and worked in the city, which was the principal hub of innovation and knowledge in the country, home to the first public library and the first hospital in the nation. By 1793, its population was estimated at around 50,000 people (Estes et al., 1997).

Despite these advances, not everything was perfect in the city. In the absence of a sewage system, human and animal waste and garbage were dumped directly into the streets. Latrines were common and not always well maintained, often leaking waste into the groundwater. The hot and humid climate, especially in summer, was ideal for the proliferation of rodents and insects, particularly mosquitoes. In addition, ships arriving from around the world constantly brought not only goods but also crew members and passengers who were carriers of diseases, many of them immigrants seeking better opportunities. Thus, the city was also the site of frequent outbreaks of a wide variety of diseases, some of which became true epidemics. Yellow fever, smallpox, typhus, dysentery, measles, and scarlet fever were common in the daily life of this post-independence colonial Philadelphia. Nevertheless, what the city would

A. Sanabria and C. Betancourt, *Cognitive Biases in Surgical Practice*,
https://doi.org/10.1007/978-3-032-20377-9_14

experience in 1793 was unprecedented and would have consequences that extended throughout the nation.

Benjamin Rush (Fig. 14.1) was born in 1745 in Byberry, Pennsylvania, near Philadelphia. The son of a prosperous family of merchants and arms manufacturers, he excelled as a student from an early age, graduating from the College of New Jersey (now Princeton University) at just 14 years old (North, 2000). His interest in medicine brought him back to Philadelphia, where he studied under John Redman, John Morgan, and William Shippen Jr., leading medical figures in the growing American colony and founders of the first medical school at the College of Philadelphia. In 1766, he left for Edinburgh, where he earned his formal medical degree two years later. He subsequently visited the leading medical centers of London and Paris before returning to Philadelphia in 1769, joining the newly founded medical school as a professor of chemistry, apparently at the request of Benjamin Franklin himself (North, 2000). The subsequent unification of the College of Philadelphia with the newly established medical school at the University of Pennsylvania made him a professor at the latter, expanding his influence in the promising American academic scene. There, he wrote the first American textbook on chemistry, the first of his many significant publications. Alongside his academic career, he developed a private medical practice, which, thanks to his knowledge and social connections, made him the personal physician of the leading political and social figures of the United States. His fervent patriotism and strong republican political convictions also led him to be one of the signers of the Independence Declaration and to participate in the Constitutional Congress in 1776. Later, during the Independence War, he was appointed as chief physician of one of the Continental Army Hospitals under George Washington's direct command. Once the war ended, he returned to Philadelphia, where he led a productive and controversial academic life (Veith, 1976).

In keeping with the era's interests and following the teachings of William Cullen, his mentor at the University of Edinburgh, Rush devoted himself to Nosology´s study, the branch of Medicine concerned with the identification, classification, categorization, description, and differentiation of diseases. Based on the knowledge available at the time, this was done according to the disease's symptoms and mechanisms thought to explain them.

Following his mentor's theories, Rush sought to deepen his work in the field, but when he tried to apply it in clinical practice, he gradually became disillusioned with the method, finding it useless for guiding the diagnosis and treatment of diseases. Nevertheless, true to his principles, he developed his own theory on the origin of diseases, abandoning Cullen's ideas. In 1789, he announced that he had discovered a new principle in medicine and that there was only one type of fever. Using the analogy of fire, he argued that just as fire could be caused by various mechanisms but was ultimately a single phenomenon, the same was true of fever, which he believed was caused by "*an irregular convulsive activity of the blood vessels*" (Kopperman, 2004). The local manifestations of diseases were related to the origin of this convulsive activity, but beyond that, they were of little importance. With a single cause, there would be a single treatment: depletive therapy, aimed at calming the "*excited*" blood vessels, based on the extensive and massive use of bloodletting and purgatives (King,

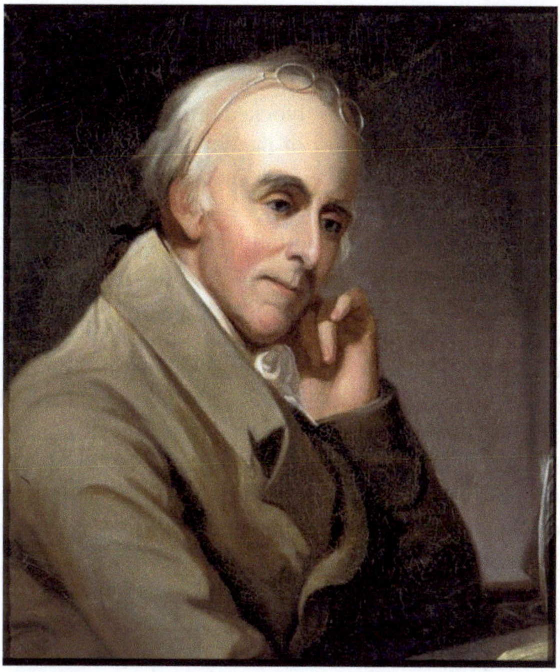

Fig. 14.1 Benjamin Rush (public domain). *Source* Charles Willson Peale—Independence National Historical Park

1991). In this context, the 1793 epidemic would provide the perfect stage for Rush to demonstrate the validity of his ideas.

The winter and spring of 1793 in Philadelphia were particularly mild and humid, so June marked the beginning of a very hot summer. As a result, mosquitoes soon infested the entire city and its surroundings. In early July, multiple merchant ships from the Caribbean arrived in the city, bringing more than 2,000 refugees escaping the Haitian Revolution. The vast majority of these, malnourished and ill, remained in Philadelphia, trying to improve their condition before continuing their journey to other destinations in the emerging United States. By the end of July, the first cases of yellow fever appeared on the city's docks. However, since these occurred among the newly arrived, they did not attract the attention of the authorities. In early August, the first cases appeared among city residents. By mid-month, the numbers had grown so fast that Rush decided to write a letter directed to the mayor of Philadelphia and the governor of Pennsylvania, warning that the city was in the early stages of an epidemic of "*intermittent bilious yellow fever*" (North, 2000). Despite rejection and ridicule from his detractors, who called him an alarmist, Rush persisted in his warnings, eventually capturing the attention of the Philadelphia College of Physicians. By August 26, when the College finally issued a statement acknowledging the epidemic and offering recommendations, the city and region were already plunged into complete chaos.

As cases and deaths multiplied uncontrollably, panic broke out. The streets filled with carts carrying the sick and dead, or with groups of healthy people trying to flee the city. Mass burials became routine. Half the city's population, including high-profile figures such as President Washington and his cabinet, escaped. Federal offices and businesses closed their doors. Neighboring towns and communities, fearful of the spread of epidemics, blocked bridges and roads, setting up checkpoints to detect and stop refugees. Most of the city's physicians had either fallen ill or fled. By the end of August, very few remained active, trying to care for thousands of patients. Rush was one of them.

Given his position and influence, Rush quickly became the leading authority in the management of the disease. At the time, the conventional treatment for fevers consisted of supportive therapy with cold drinks, a light diet, rest, and very mild doses of laxatives. Rush began his clinical practice with these measures, but after discouraging initial results (four of his first five patients treated during the pandemic died), he abandoned them in favor of his own ideas. The extensive use of purgatives and, especially, massive bloodletting became routine. By mid-September, the recommendation was to remove at least four liters of blood from patients within no more than five days (Rush, 1974). In his view, the human body contained at least 11 liters of blood and up to 9 could be removed, so there was no problem with this practice. Rush entered a state of exaltation rarely seen, treating more than 100 patients a day and turning his home into a clinic. So much blood was drawn that his garden became a foul-smelling place, swarming with flies.

Despite the worse outcomes, Rush proclaimed the success of his therapy, promoting it in newspapers, advertisements, and pamphlets, and criticizing anyone who did not adhere to it. When he himself fell ill, he did not hesitate to treat himself according to his own methods. His recovery was the final proof he needed to convince himself of the validity of his theory. Despite his self-proclaimed success, most of the region's medical community, including the College of Physicians, rejected his methods, calling him a "*murderer*" and accusing him of using bloodletting "*fit for horses*" (North, 2000). When warnings went unheeded, he was expelled from the College of Physicians and even threatened with criminal charges. In response, he claimed that his methods had been revealed to him by God himself, of whom he was merely an instrument, and that in the face of the doctors' rejection, he had the gratitude of the many people saved thanks to his method (Shryock, 1971).

With the arrival of cold air at the end of autumn and the beginning of winter, the mosquitoes disappeared and, as a result, the pandemic ended. The return to normal life in the city brought an assessment of consequences. The numbers were more than terrible. More than five thousand people (about 10% of the city's population) had died. During this devastation, there was another number that could not be ignored. Despite the grim prognosis of yellow fever, it had only been particularly deadly when Rush's recommendations for massive bloodletting were adopted. This reality was so undeniable and striking that a well-known journalist of the time wrote that Rush had made "*one of the greatest discoveries to contribute to the depopulation of earth*" (North, 2000).

When analyzing this story, it is easy to think of Benjamin Rush as a deeply disturbed individual whose position and connections at the time allowed him to exert such a dangerous influence. History is full of similar examples. However, Rush's case does not seem to fit this description, as he was one of the most important figures in the birth of academic medicine in the United States, and his contributions and publications in medical education and psychiatry justify this status. Several medical schools bear his name, and to this day, he is the only person to whom the American Medical Association has erected a statue. Titles such as the "*Hippocrates of Pennsylvania*" or the "*father of modern psychiatry*" are well deserved. Nevertheless, this episode is an undeniable stain on his brilliant career. The question that arises is how someone so brilliant in other areas of medicine could make such a significant mistake, and why he remained committed to it even when the results were not as expected. The answer likely lies in the overconfidence bias.

Definition

Overconfidence bias is the flawed thinking process by which one systematically overestimates one's own abilities, knowledge, and the accuracy of one's judgments and reasoning. In other words, it is the belief that one is more intelligent, more capable, more knowledgeable, more logical, and more rational than one actually is. Essentially, it is the belief that one is better in every respect than reality dictates.

By the time the 1793 pandemic began, Rush was perhaps the most influential and recognized medical figure in Philadelphia. His publications and contributions to structuring the University of Pennsylvania's medical school gave him great influence in the nascent American academic scene. His social standing and connections had made him the trusted physician of many of the most important figures in the emerging nation. In turn, his discoveries in Nosology´s field and his unifying theory of fever could only have come from someone with deep confidence in his own abilities. The implementation of these measures with the arrival of the pandemic was nothing more than a logical action in his reasoning. His dissemination of these ideas, his staunch defense when deserved criticism arose, the outlandish arguments used to defend them, and especially his confidence in having applied them to himself when faced the disease, all speak of a person deeply convinced that he was right. The unfortunate consequences are already known to us.

History

Overconfidence in judgments and reasoning was first described by Stuart Oskamp in 1965 (Oskamp, 1965). In his research, he provided a group of psychologists with sequential information about a hypothetical patient. After each round of data, they were asked to answer a multiple-choice questionnaire regarding their assessments. Each answer had to be accompanied by a percentage indicating how confident they were in the accuracy of their statement. With each additional round of information, the process was repeated (the questions and answer options always remained the same).

After four rounds of data, the experiment concluded. Upon analyzing the results, two things became obvious: first, the participants systematically overestimated the certainty of their answers; second, additional information did not increase the accuracy of the answers, but it did substantially increase the participants' confidence in them. In other words, more information led to greater overconfidence.

Baruch Fischhoff, Paul Slovic, and Sarah Lichtenstein later developed a series of studies that allowed for the definition of bias (Fischhoff et al., 1977). Variations of a central experiment were conducted in different scenarios and situations, asking participants to answer general knowledge questions (usually multiple choice with only two options) and to rate how confident they were in the accuracy of their answers. Systematically, the accuracy of the answers was always overestimated. Regardless of other variables (participants' level of education, question difficulty, expectations and risks involved, etc.), the results were always the same.

Multiple subsequent studies have repeatedly confirmed the findings of Fischhoff and Lichtenstein. Among these, the study by Justin Kruger and David Dunning is particularly important; they later demonstrated that the less someone knows about a subject, the greater their confidence in their apparent (but in reality, nonexistent) ability and/or knowledge (Kruger & Dunning, 1999).

Impact

Overconfidence bias directly affects self-assessment of knowledge, skills, and abilities. In this sense, it is expected to impact on all facets of human life. Among the most important are:

At the Personal Level:

1. **Inadequate decision-making:** Believing oneself to be more capable and knowledgeable than one actually is directs to make decisions quicker without considering all available information and without evaluating the specific details of each situation. This results in poor decisions, especially in complex scenarios and circumstances that require more careful and thorough analysis.
2. **Increased risk-taking:** By overestimating one's abilities and knowledge, the challenges and difficulties inherent in each situation are underestimated and reckless decisions are made without assessing their consequences, thereby increasing the likelihood of errors.
3. **Difficulty in learning:** A fundamental condition for acquiring new skills and knowledge is the ability to recognize one's own limitations and weaknesses in order to address and overcome them. This bias hinders this process, limiting opportunities for growth and future improvement.
4. **Lack of social interaction and empathy:** By overvaluing one's own judgments and conclusions, there is a reduced tendency to listen to others, accept constructive criticism, and consider alternative perspectives, due to the belief that one's

own view is the only correct and/or appropriate one. Additionally, thoughts such as "*I should have known*," "*I would have acted differently*," or "*that wouldn't have happened to me*" make it more difficult to understand others' problems and to offer help.

At the Collective Level:

1. **Suppression of dissent:** Excessive confidence in leaders or the majority opinion creates an environment where questioning decisions and/or opinions is seen as disloyalty or weakness. As a result, members who have doubts or contradictory information self-censor to avoid disrupting the apparent harmony of the group, eliminating necessary debate and constructive criticism that enrich the decision-making process.
2. **Possibility of catastrophic events:** When most people involved in carrying out a complex task or achieving a goal systematically overestimate their abilities and underestimate the risks, small failures can sequentially accumulate, with each new error magnifying the previous one and snowballing into serious situations and disasters. Catastrophes such as the sinking of the Titanic or the Chernobyl explosion can be explained by this phenomenon.

Examples in Medical and Surgical Practice

Physicians, especially surgeons, due to the nature of their training and the demands of professional practice, are particularly prone to overconfidence. In this regard, it is foreseeable that the effects of this bias are frequent and varied. Among the most significant are:

1. **Erroneous or delayed diagnoses**: Being overly confident in their knowledge, a surgeon may become convinced of a certain diagnosis, overlooking other possibilities and failing to request additional tests that would confirm their hypothesis and rule out other options, regardless of how atypical the case may be. For example, a surgeon evaluating a woman with mild lower abdominal pain at mid-cycle may, who without further investigation diagnose painful ovulation and miss an atypical case of acute appendicitis.
2. **Underestimation of intraoperative surgical risks**: Confident in their skills and ability to manage any situation that may arise during surgery, surgeons may downplay the inherent risks of a procedure or dismiss the possibility of intraoperative complications. For example, a surgeon who proceeds to operate on a patient with a borderline resectable cancer without adequate preoperative assessment because "*I am capable of removing it*."
3. **Denial of complications**: Confident that a surgery was performed perfectly, early symptoms and signs of complications that would allow for prompt diagnosis and timely treatment may be overlooked. For example, a surgeon who ignores the early signs of peritonitis after a laparoscopic cholecystectomy because "*that surgery was perfect*."

4. **Failure to seek a second opinion or request assistance**: Confidence in one's own abilities makes surgeons reluctant to seek help from colleagues, which can be detrimental in complex or high-risk cases that would benefit from a multidisciplinary approach. For example, a surgeon who proceeds to operate alone on a complex patient, disregarding the assistance of other relevant specialists, because "*I can do this all by myself*."
5. **Rejection of therapeutic advances**: Confident in the success of their treatments throughout their professional career, a surgeon may become resistant to adopting new and improved therapeutic options that could reduce or prevent morbidity and decrease risks. For example, a surgeon who dismisses the use of a particular immunotherapy in cancer management because "*I have always operated on these patients and they do well.*"

How to Avoid Falling into the Bias

1. **Acknowledgements the existence of bias:** Understanding and accepting the presence of bias is a first step toward overcoming it. In this sense, although it may be difficult, accept that one is not as capable, intelligent, wise or logical as one believes.
2. **Adopt a growth mindset:** Instead of believing that you know everything or that your skills are at their peak, assume that there is always room to learn and improve. This fosters humility and enhances the willingness to seek new knowledge and abilities.
3. **Seek feedback and diverse opinions:** Surround yourself with people who provide sincere and honest feedback on your ideas, plans, and skills. Consider their perspectives, especially if they differ from your own. Avoid flatterers.
4. **Practice intellectual humility:** Recognize that it is impossible to know or do everything. Accept that your knowledge and beliefs are incomplete and may be incorrect. Understand that skills can always be improved. This attitude will help you be more receptive to learning and less likely to defend your own positions blindly.
5. **Keep a record of predictions:** Write down your predictions and estimates, and once the outcome is known, compare them to what actually happened. Reviewing past errors leads to reduced overconfidence in your knowledge and reasoning. In turn, analyzing mistakes will help you better calibrate future judgments.
6. **Use the "pre-mortem" strategy:** Before making any important decision, regardless of how confident you are, imagine that the decision has resulted in a spectacular failure and then write down all the possible reasons why this could have happened. This tactic forces you to consider all the risks and potential failures that bias might be concealing.

References

Estes, J. W., Smith, B. G., & Smith, B. G. (1997). *A melancholy scene of devastation: The public response to the 1793 Philadelphia yellow fever epidemic*. College of Physicians of Philadelphia and the Library Company of Philadelphia. https://books.google.com.co/books?id=MRfIwih28gIC

Fischhoff, B., Slovic, P., & Lichtenstein, S. (1977). Knowing with certainty: The appropriateness of extreme confidence. *Journal of Experimental Psychology: Human Perception and Performance, 3*(4), 552–564. https://doi.org/10.1037/0096-1523.3.4.552

King, L. S. (1991). *Transformations in American medicine: From Benjamin Rush to William Osler*. Johns Hopkins University Press.

Kopperman, P. E. (2004). "Venerate the Lancet": Benjamin Rush's yellow fever therapy in context. *Bulletin of the History of Medicine, 78*(3), 539–574. https://doi.org/10.1353/bhm.2004.0126

Kruger, J., & Dunning, D. (1999). Unskilled and unaware of it: How difficulties in recognizing one's own incompetence lead to inflated self-assessments. *Journal of Personality and Social Psychology, 77*(6), 1121–1134. https://doi.org/10.1037//0022-3514.77.6.1121

North, R. L. (2000). Benjamin Rush, MD: Assassin or beloved healer? *Proceedings (Baylor University. Medical Center), 13*(1), 45–49. https://doi.org/10.1080/08998280.2000.11927641

Oskamp, S. (1965). Overconfidence in case-study judgments. *Journal of Consulting Psychology, 29*(3), 261–265. https://doi.org/10.1037/h0022125

Rush, B. (1974). *An account of the bilious remitting yellow fever, as it appeared in the city of Philadelphia, in the year 1793*. Thomas Dobson. https://collections.nlm.nih.gov/bookviewer?PID=nlm:nlmuid-2569009R-bk

Shryock, R. H. (1971). The medical reputation of Benjamin Rush: Contrasts over two centuries. *Bulletin of the History of Medicine, 45*(6), 507–552.

Veith, I. (1976). Benjamin Rush and the beginnings of American Medicine. *Western Journal of Medicine, 125*(1), 17–27.

References

[illegible]

Chapter 15
Omission Bias. Laparotomy in Abdominal Trauma

The Problem

The introduction of anesthesia in 1846 and antisepsis in 1867 paved the way for safer abdominal surgery. By this time, abdominal wounds were common in armed conflicts, and since the American Civil War, their management was limited to keeping the patient at rest, controlling temperature, removing penetrating objects, controlling external bleeding, and closing the wound while maintaining fasting, general supportive measures, and hydrating enemas. As expected, death was the most frequent outcome. In search of better results, George Goodfellow, an American surgeon who served in the Spanish-American War, and George Alexander Otis, who recorded statistics from the American Civil War, had challenged this approach, but their findings remained largely unrecognized (Senn, 1900).

By 1890, two schools of thought existed among military surgeons: (Bennett, 1991) the interventionists, who advocated early laparotomy, and the abstentionists, who opposed it. The interventionists were led by James Marion Sims, an American surgeon and one of the fathers of gynecology. The abstentionist group was led by Jean Jacques Paul Reclus, who argued that abdominal wounds were self-limiting without treatment, a view supported by surgical experience in previous wars (Chinese Japanese (1894), Spanish-American (1898)). Although initially in favor of intervention, Sir William MacCormac ("Sir William MacCormac," 1883), an Irish surgeon who served in the Franco-Prussian War in 1870 and had demonstrated lower mortality with early laparotomy compared to the near-total mortality of conservative management, changed his opinion after returning from South Africa, where he served in the Boer War, to the extent that the famous MacCormac aphorism was coined: "*In this war a man wounded in the abdomen dies if he is operated upon and remains alive if he is left in peace.*" Given his fame and reputation, this policy became popular and was maintained in subsequent conflicts (the French war in Morocco and the Balkan Wars) until the Russo-Japanese War of 1904. At that time, Frederick Treves (Gibbs, 1992), an English surgeon renowned for performing the first appendectomy in the

A. Sanabria and C. Betancourt, *Cognitive Biases in Surgical Practice*,
https://doi.org/10.1007/978-3-032-20377-9_15

United Kingdom and for being Queen Victoria's surgeon, strongly reinforced this position, stating in his Manual of Operative Surgery: "*Experience has shown that indiscriminate irrigation of the abdominal cavity does more harm than good, and that 'evisceration' and rough handling of the damaged intestines is dangerous.*"

Despite the widespread acceptance of this approach, some dissenting voices began to emerge in favor of intervention, such as Vera Gedroitz (Bennett, 1992), a princess and the first Russian female surgeon, who demonstrated the value of early laparotomy in the Russian front, leading to its adoption by the entire Russian army. Although her results were published, they were ignored for a long time, due to her association with the Bolsheviks and her status as a lesbian in a conservative society.

At that time, despite emerging evidence, many surgeons remained convinced that rest, fasting, and analgesics were sufficient treatment for these wounds. Among the reasons for defending this position was the belief that all intestinal wounds were fatal, making any procedure futile (Fig. 15.1). Additionally, reports from the Official History of The War in South Africa 1899–1902 (Maurice & Grant, 2016) mentioned some successful cases of conservative management, which were widely publicized by surviving soldiers, even though most weapons used in that war fired low-energy projectiles that did not penetrate the abdominal wall. Finally, there was the notion that surgical management could not be performed under battlefield conditions due to the risk of infection, despite the well-known successful experience of Gedroitz. Underlying all this was a nihilistic belief that laparotomy carried too many risks, so it was considered better to avoid it. However, data such as a 20% reduction in mortality and the explanation that failures of the interventional approach were due to delayed surgeries began to emerge, contradicting this belief.

In this setting, Owen Richards, a British surgeon under the command of Sir Cuthbert Sidney Wallace, was one of the pioneers of the interventional approach during the early years of the First World War, when he instituted mandatory laparotomy for the management of abdominal wounds, even against the orders of his superiors (Asensio et al., 2016). Initially, other surgeons attempted surgery with disastrous results and subsequently abandoned the effort, a situation that was only reversed after autopsies of deceased soldiers demonstrated that surgery would have been the only chance for survival. These findings prompted surgeons to take a more active stance and stop watching soldiers bleed to death under the observation of officers. Thus, in 1918, Sidney Wallace, a British surgeon from St Thomas's Hospital in London, published his book War Surgery of the Abdomen (Wallace, 1918), in which he described his experience with early surgical treatment of abdominal wounds during the First World War and the improved outcomes with laparotomy. Among his observations, he highlighted the streaks of bad luck that military surgeons had to face, which had a demoralizing effect and could lead to the belief that perhaps a watchful waiting approach was preferable. He also noted that failing to consider the overall pattern of failures relative to the number of successes could increase the perception of providing the wrong treatment. Furthermore, he mentioned the ongoing debate between groups: while interventionists argued that death was generally due to hemorrhage, which could be controlled surgically, conservatives believed that the cause of death was peritonitis, which was aggravated by laparotomy as it prevented the intestines from sealing the

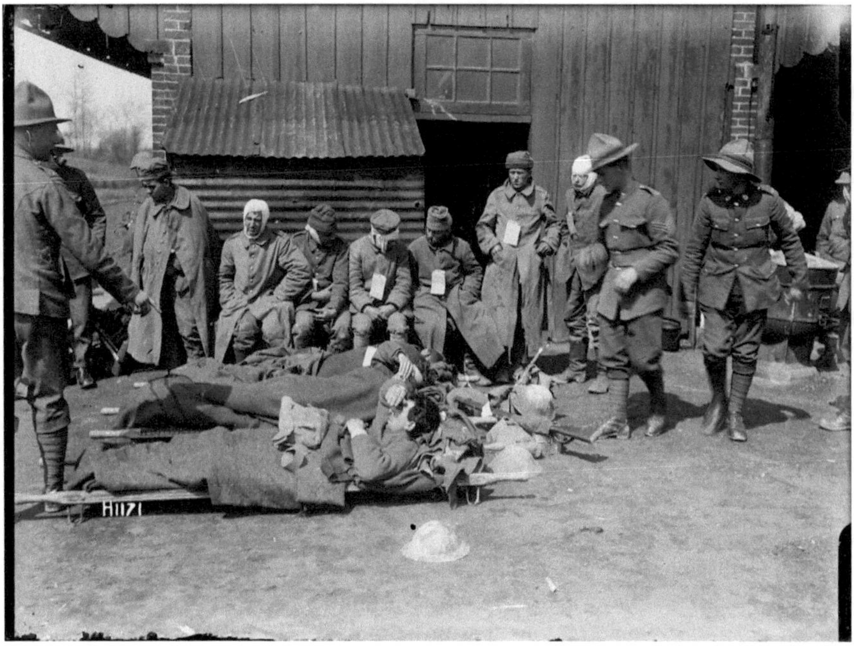

Fig. 15.1 Wound care units in the First World War (public domain) https://natlib.govt.nz/

perforations themselves. He also cited the differences in outcomes between civilian and military casualties, along with growing criticism from civilian authorities who could not distinguish between the two and demanded lower mortality rates. Despite all this, it was not until 1924, long after the end of the First World War, that surgical attitudes toward penetrating abdominal trauma began to change, thanks to the advocacy of surgeons such as the German Victor Schmieden and the New Zealander Douglas Jolly.

The history of trauma surgery contains many examples that can be attributed to the effect of omission bias. One only need to recall Billroth, the father of gastrointestinal surgery, who stated: "*The surgeon who attempts to suture a cardiac wound will lose the respect of his colleagues,*" a view that for years closed the door to beneficial interventions (Absolon & McGoon, 1983). The example described above of laparotomy in abdominal trauma illustrates the power exerted by omission bias in surgical decision-making. It is easy to imagine a surgeon facing a critical situation requiring a fast decision that could have disastrous consequences but might also save a life, such as a patient with a penetrating abdominal wound at the time. It is not difficult to deduce the thoughts that might have crossed his mind in those moments: if he operates and succeeds, he will be a hero. But if he fails, the adverse outcome will be attributed to his intervention, and he will be judged and criticized by his colleagues for having done something that may have contributed to the negative result. On the other hand, if for some reason he decides not to operate and the patient survives, he will be praised for his insight and clinical judgment; but if the patient dies, his omission will likely be accepted and interpreted as the natural course of the condition, where any intervention would have been futile. It is unlikely he will be blamed. In this scenario, the second option naturally seems preferable, even though available data showed that intervention, despite its inherent risks, was the better choice. Surgeons who chose to operate (action), despite achieving better overall outcomes, were initially held responsible for fatal results and labeled as reckless and imprudent. In contrast, surgeons who avoided laparotomy (omission) maintained their authority and status, even though most patients died and they later changed their approach. The price paid for their omission was low. The consequences for the patients, however, were dramatically different.

Definition

Omission bias is defined as the tendency, when faced with a decision, to prefer inaction (omission) over action (commission), as people attribute greater weight to the consequences of actions than to those of omissions, even when the frequency of both is similar. Some reasons that favor omission in decision-making include ignorance, the desire for good intentions, and convenience, as omission requires less effort compared to commission, which is often premeditated, ill-intentioned, and demands greater cognitive effort (Ritov & Baron, 1990).

In moral terms, there seem to be more ways to justify not acting than to justify deliberate action, although there are cases where this norm must be carefully evaluated in relation to the consequences and the actors involved (Thomson, 1976). Some authors have suggested that omission, in addition to being a bias, has a rational, strategic component, implying that people know omission protects them from being held accountable for negative outcomes, in contrast to action (Hallsworth et al., 2015).

There is a heuristic based on the idea that acting and causing negative consequences is worse than not acting and having the same consequences (omission is neutral, while action can be judged as positive or negative), and this is used in daily life. However, this idea is based on the premise that the consequences of action or omission are identical. When this premise changes, even if action yields better outcomes than omission, the heuristic continues to be used, leading to wrong decisions (Baron & Ritov, 1994).

On the other hand, omission is perceived as a protection against the moral responsibilities of a decision, as a form of loss aversion. If one does not actively participate in a decision, it is impossible to assign any degree of blame if the outcome is adverse. Conversely, if one acts and the result is unexpected, this may be seen as a loss (Ritov & Baron, 1999).

Another alternative explanation relates omission to the *status quo*. If an action is omitted, it is not possible for unexpected consequences to be attributed to anyone; it is the fault of the system, nature, or customs. If one acts and this action has consequences, causally it is possible to assign them to the action taken (Ritov & Baron, 1992).

It has also been proposed that omission bias is related to social norms, where the fear of being judged by the community favors inaction over an action that could potentially yield better results but is disapproved by the environment (the bad Samaritan).

It has been shown that omission bias increases with age, but differences related to cultural or educational context have not been explored.

History

In 1967, Philippa Foot (Foot, 2002), a British philosopher, addressed the discussion of the "*doctrine of double effect*," which describes that certain actions, with good intentions, can have foreseeable adverse consequences (collateral damage) that are acceptable and morally justifiable, in the sense that they were not done with the intention to harm. In her explanation, Foot argues that the acceptance of these consequences is based on the idea that if I intend to cause harm, this harm is morally attributable to my intention (action). Conversely, if harm occurs because of an action without the intention to harm, it is not morally attributable to the decision (omission). Among her examples, she included what would later be called "*the trolley problem*," an ethical experiment in which a train conductor who has lost the brakes must decide at a track split whether to run over five people on one side or just one person on the other (Thomson, 1976). This gave rise to a broad ethical discussion but established the foundations that were later used to define omission bias.

In 1986, David Sugarman proposed the problem of euthanasia (Sugarman, 1986), in which he morally evaluated the attitudes of a hypothetical physician toward active euthanasia (administering some therapy to accelerate death) compared to passive euthanasia (withholding therapies that would prolong life). Although the final consequence was the same, the patient's death, examples in which physicians opted for active euthanasia were judged more negatively, assigned greater responsibility, and their actions were considered outside the standards of the medical profession.

In 1990, Ilana Ritov and Jonathan Baron designed the vaccination problem (Ritov & Baron, 1990) to evaluate omission bias. Their example was based on known data about the risk and effectiveness of the DPT vaccine, which showed that its effectiveness was greater in relation to mortality and that there had been cases in which the vaccine manufacturer had been taken to court for the few cases where the vaccine caused an adverse event, but there had never been a lawsuit for the number of cases where the vaccine failed to prevent the disease. The authors demonstrated that subjects are reluctant to vaccinate due to adverse events, even though these are far fewer than the potential deaths prevented by the vaccine.

In 1991, Mark Spranca, Elisa Minsk, and Jonathan Baron from the University of Pennsylvania (Spranca et al., 1991) applied this concept to decision-making with the famous "*tennis tournament*" experiment, considered as evidence for the existence of omission bias. In a tennis tournament, the two finalists face each other in a match, where one has a clear athletic advantage over the other. However, the disadvantaged player knows about the other's food allergy. At a dinner before the final match, the food options include the allergenic product, which the more skilled player is unaware of, but the less skilled player knows. In this situation, the disadvantaged tennis player has three options: first, to recommend the sauce with the allergen (action); second, knowing the food contains the allergen, to remain silent and let the opponent order it (omission); and third, even if the opponent has chosen another dish, to persuade him to choose the one with the allergen, knowing it will cause an adverse reaction. The results of the experiment showed that the omission option was judged as less blameworthy (as if actively lying were somehow considered worse than concealing the truth).

Impact

At the Personal Level:

1. **Inaction as a Psychological Shield.** Omission bias affects risk perception toward others, reinforcing the idea that by not participating in an action, one is more morally protected ("*I simply found myself in that situation; I am not to blame for what happened*") or requires less emotional burden ("*better to leave things as they are*").
2. **Moral Perceptions in Choices About Inaction.** Classic examples include the decision not to vaccinate in response to existing adverse risks, which are much lower than the probability of contracting the disease in the absence of vaccination. Another example is organ donation, where omitting the decision to donate (leaving the responsibility for decision to others) feels morally more justified than actively deciding not to donate (self-respectability).

At the Collective Level:

1. **Harsher Judgments for Action Versus Inaction.** In addition, the bias can delay decision-making and compromise future outcomes, as when a large-scale financial intervention is needed (liquidating an investment that is generating losses), but is postponed due to uncertainty about the outcome. In general, people are more likely to judge more harshly and compensate less those who act compared to those who refrain from acting.
2. **Defaults and Inaction Exploited in Purchasing Behavior.** In purchasing decisions, strategies focused on omission bias (you will miss the benefit, you will have to pay more next time) are used to prevent the customer from deciding, as occurs with the suspension of continuous renewal services. In other cases, unsolicited services (a meal, a ticket to an event) are added and charged along with the initial purchase, taking advantage of the tendency toward inaction so that people do not reject these add-ons. Another approach involves automating

certain steps (default options), such as pre-filled data entry, which ensures the action flow continues by leveraging the tendency toward inaction. In cases of financial crisis when staff reduction decisions are required, stopping hiring is an easier option to accept than having to lay off employees.

Examples in Medical and Surgical Practice

In surgery, there are a significant number of examples of omission bias.

1. **Avoidance of Intervention Despite Potential Benefit**. The surgeon may choose not to perform high-risk surgery compared to conservative management, even when the surgery offers benefits that outweigh expectant management. For example, a transplant surgery in a patient with chronic kidney disease carries potential risks of death similar to those of long-term maintenance with dialysis, but with clear improvements in cardiovascular risk and quality of life.
2. **End-of-Life Choices Shaped by Inaction Preference**. In cases of critical illness requiring advanced life support measures, and where the disease course is ominous and progressing toward death, it is easier to decide not to initiate life support measures (omission) than to withdraw them once started (commission) (Ursin, 2019).
3. **Resistance to Protocols Due to Rare Adverse Outcomes**. When implementing a surgical policy (trauma triage to select patients for immediate treatment) that may yield beneficial results for the majority, there is resistance due to potential negative effects (a triaged-out patient with a severe condition who dies), regardless of how infrequent these are.
4. **Differential Attribution of Responsibility in Complications**. When a complication is reviewed in a morbidity and mortality meeting, responsibility is more often attributed to the surgeon when it results from an action (for example, in a difficult cholecystectomy, the surgeon decides to proceed and causes a bile duct injury) than when it results from an omission (in a difficult cholecystectomy, the surgeon decides to abort the procedure, but the patient dies from biliary sepsis).
5. **Greater Accountability for Action Than Inaction**. When facing an administrative situation related to inappropriate use of resources, greater blame is assigned in cases where a resource is frequently used (action) in situations where there is no benefit (recommending and performing a treatment such as arthroscopy in cases of osteoarthritis, where there is no evidence-based justification) than in cases where the same treatment is not rejected (omission) (performing an arthroscopy in osteoarthritis because another colleague or the health system had already requested the procedure).
6. **Nonmaleficence and the Preference for Omission**. Even in ethical discussions, the principle of "*primum non nocere*" emphasizes avoiding the risk of action, favoring omission as justifiable (Aberegg et al., 2005).

How to Avoid Falling into Bias

1. **Awareness of the existence of the bias:** As with all biases, being aware of them helps to recognize and potentially avoid them.
2. **Actively compare the consequences of inaction with those of action:** Assess what happens if a particular intervention is not performed and what its risks are, comparing them with the benefits and risks of undertaking the action.
3. **Use risk–benefit assessment tools:** These allow for a better understanding of the real consequences of action and omission, helping to reduce the effect of bias. These include cost–benefit analyses, decision trees, best–worst scenario strategies, etc.
4. **Conduct counterfactual analysis:** Systematically evaluate what the hypothetical outcomes would have been if a different decision had been made. This allows each situation to be placed in a real context, reducing the tendency to blame adverse outcomes on action and to excuse omission.
5. **Use reframing:** Since inaction is considered morally less distressing than action, it is possible to redesign or invert the framing of options. For example, if omission is noted regarding the use of a more invasive but more effective diagnostic method (digital rectal exam) with similar risks to another (PSA blood test), the options can be presented by making the PSA method the active alternative, emphasizing the number of false positives leading to unnecessary surgery and the consequent risk of impotence, leaving the digital rectal exam as the passive option.
6. **Show evidence that the decision to remain inactive was made voluntarily:** This strategy can help omission to be avoided or mitigated. If a surgeon decides not to operate on a patient with abdominal pain who has clear clinical signs of an acute abdomen and the patient has an adverse outcome (death), demonstrating that the decision not to operate was made voluntarily and rationally (it was early morning, there were no other concurrent cases, the operating room was available) mitigates omission bias by increasing the likelihood of morally holding the individual accountable for their decision (DeScioli et al., 2011).

References

Aberegg, S. K., Haponik, E. F., & Terry, P. B. (2005). Omission bias and decision making in pulmonary and critical care medicine. *Chest, 128*(3), 1497–1505. https://doi.org/10.1378/chest.128.3.1497

Absolon, K. B., & McGoon, D. C. (1983). Theodor Billroth and cardiac surgery. *The Journal of Thoracic and Cardiovascular Surgery, 86* (3), 451–452. https://doi.org/10.1016/S0022-5223(19)39162-7

Asensio, J. A., Petrone, P., Ogun, O. A., Perez-Alonso, A. J., Wagner, M., Bertellotti, R., Phillips, B. J., & Udekwu, A. O. (2016). Laparotomy: The conquering of the abdomen and the historical journey of pancreatic and duodenal injuries. *Journal of Trauma and Acute Care Surgery, 80*(6), 1023–1031. https://doi.org/10.1097/TA.0000000000001010

Baron, J., & Ritov, I. (1994). Reference points and omission bias. *Organizational Behavior and Human Decision Processes, 59*(3), 475–498. https://doi.org/10.1006/obhd.1994.1070
Bennett, J. D. (1991). Abdominal surgery in war–the early story. *Journal of the Royal Society of Medicine, 84*(9), 554–557. https://doi.org/10.1177/014107689108400917
Bennett, J. D. (1992). Princess Vera Gedroits: Military surgeon, poet, and author. *BMJ, 305*(6868), 1532–1534. https://doi.org/10.1136/bmj.305.6868.1532
DeScioli, P., Bruening, R., & Kurzban, R. (2011). The omission effect in moral cognition: Toward a functional explanation. *Evolution and Human Behavior, 32*(3), 204–215. https://doi.org/10.1016/j.evolhumbehav.2011.01.003
Foot, P. (2002). The problem of abortion and the doctrine of the double effect*. In P. Foot (Ed.), *Virtues and vices: And other essays in moral philosophy* (p. 0). https://doi.org/10.1093/0199252866.003.0002
Gibbs, D. D. (1992). Sir Frederick Treves: Surgeon, author and medical historian. *Journal of the Royal Society of Medicine, 85*(9), 565–569. https://doi.org/10.1177/014107689208500919
Hallsworth, M., List, J., Metcalfe, R., & Vlaev, I. (2015). The making of Homo Honoratus: From omission to commission.
Maurice, M. G. F., & Grant, C. M. H. (2016). *Official history of the war in South Africa 1899–1902 compiled by the direction of his majesty's government volume two maps*. Naval & Military Press. https://books.google.com.co/books?id=cWUVMQAACAAJ
Ritov, I., & Baron, J. (1992). Status-quo and omission biases. *Journal of risk and uncertainty, 5*(1), 49–61.
Ritov, I., & Baron, J. (1990). Reluctance to vaccinate: Omission bias and ambiguity. *Journal of Behavioral Decision Making, 3*(4), 263–277. https://doi.org/10.1002/bdm.3960030404
Ritov, I., & Baron, J. (1999). Protected values and omission bias. *Organizational Behavior and Human Decision Processes, 79*(2), 79–94. https://doi.org/10.1006/obhd.1999.2839
Senn, N. (1900). *Medico-surgical aspects of the Spanish American War*. American Med. Assoc. Press. https://books.google.com.co/books?id=Mqhb0QEACAAJ
Sir William MacCormac. (1883). *Journal of the American medical association, I* (12), 370–371. https://doi.org/10.1001/jama.1883.02390120018006
Spranca, M., Minsk, E., & Baron, J. (1991). *Omission and commission in judgment and choice*. Elsevier Science. https://doi.org/10.1016/0022-1031(91)90011-T
Sugarman, D. B. (1986). Active versus passive euthanasia: An attributional analysis. *Journal of Applied Social Psychology, 16*(1), 60–76. https://doi.org/10.1111/j.1559-1816.1986.tb02278.x
Thomson, J. J. (1976). Killing, letting die, and the trolley problem. *The Monist, 59*(2), 204–217. https://doi.org/10.5840/monist197659224
Ursin, L. (2019). Withholding and withdrawing life-sustaining treatment: Ethically equivalent? *American Journal of Bioethics, 19*(3), 10–20. https://doi.org/10.1080/15265161.2018.1561961
Wallace, C. S. (1918). *War surgery of the abdomen.* J. & A. Churchill. https://books.google.com.co/books?id=jnTy2xD88OcC

Chapter 16
Bandwagon Effect. The Rise and Fall of the Adjustable Gastric Band

The Problem

Obesity arises when energy intake exceeds expenditure over a prolonged period. Despite the apparent simplicity of this equation, the factors involved (genetic, metabolic, environmental, economic, social, cultural, behavioral, etc.) are numerous, diverse and complex, affecting both sides of the equation and making obesity a multifaceted and difficult problem to address. Defined as an excess of body fat (Hensrud & Klein, 2006), different surrogate measures are used to assess it, since direct measurement is complex and impractical. Among these, the most widely accepted and used is the body mass index (BMI), which is currently the standard for its assessment and diagnosis. Thus, obesity is defined as a BMI equal to or greater than 30, and morbid or severe obesity as a BMI equal to or greater than 40 (NIH, 2001).

Beyond the structural, psychological, and social problems associated with excess weight, obesity is linked to an increased risk of developing multiple and severe comorbidities, such as hypertension, diabetes mellitus, dyslipidemia, coronary artery disease, sleep apnea, fatty liver disease, certain types of cancer, etc., which are among the leading causes of non-traumatic death worldwide. The prevalence of obesity has increased alarmingly over the past 40 years. By 2003, it was estimated that 32.2% of the United States population was obese (Ogden et al., 2006). Similar studies reported that approximately 9.8% of the global population was obese in 2005. Even more concerning, based on previous trends, it is expected that by 2030 there will be around 573 million obese individuals (Kelly et al., 2008). Thus, obesity has become a global epidemic with serious economic and social consequences (Powers et al., 2007). In terms of costs alone, obesity represents a greater health expenditure than other diseases considered more severe, such as cancer, not to mention other aspects that are more difficult to measure, such as reduced work capacity or years of productive life lost due to premature death (Finkelstein et al., 2003).

For this reason, it was necessary to design strategies to address this growing problem in all its aspects, from prevention to treatment. Thus, in 2001, the United

A. Sanabria and C. Betancourt, *Cognitive Biases in Surgical Practice*,
https://doi.org/10.1007/978-3-032-20377-9_16

States Public Health Service, the National Institutes of Health, the Centers for Disease Control and Prevention and the Office of the Surgeon General of the U.S. Department of Health published a joint document calling on all stakeholders (citizens and physicians involved in patient care; food production and distribution chains; scientific research centers, etc.) to design and implement alternatives to address the problem at every stage (NIH, 2001).

At the treatment level, among all available options, no strategy has proven more effective than bariatric surgery. Although its origins date back to the 1950s, these procedures remained largely ignored for many years until the 1990s, with the emergence of obesity as an epidemic, when they began to play an increasing role in disease management. Despite the multiple procedures available, their varying scopes and objectives and the heterogeneity in selection and implementation criteria, bariatric surgery is the best available strategy for treating obesity, especially in its more advanced stages, due to its effects on the percentage of excess weight lost, long-term sustainability, improvement and resolution of comorbidities, increased quality of life, cost-effectiveness, etc (Dumon & Murayama, 2011).

Despite its undeniable benefits, by the 1990s there were multiple concerns regarding the long-term impact and consequences (primarily nutritional and metabolic) that these procedures could have once obesity was resolved. Given that the available procedures at the time were irreversible, the development of a reversible technique was the dream of all surgeons involved in obesity treatment. The idea of a gastric band that could restrict food intake without altering the stomach's configuration was conceived by Lawrence Wilkinson in the early 1970s, based on his experiments with dogs. Wilkinson, a successful surgeon and researcher from New Mexico (USA), began by placing a polypropylene mesh around a 36 Fr. tube positioned along the lesser curvature of the stomach, aiming to exclude the greater curvature and the rest of the stomach from the passage of food. Building on his animal experience and later refining the technique in humans, he developed and patented a preformed mesh for this purpose in 1983 (Wilkinson, 1980). However, the difficulty in creating a sufficiently small gastric reservoir led to the idea being quickly abandoned. Despite this initial failure, Wilkinson and Anthony Peloso continued their work and were the first to place a two-centimeter, non-adjustable Marlex mesh around the upper third of the stomach in 1978, limiting the lumen to the minimum size required to allow passage of a 36 Fr. tube (Wilkinson & Peloso, 1981). This concept was much more promising and quickly gained interest, with surgeons in Norway, Australia, Sweden, and other parts of the United States reporting similar experiences with minor variations in the type and configuration of the material used for the band (always non-adjustable) (Steffen, 2008).

Despite the initial enthusiasm, short-term results proved discouraging. The challenges of creating a small gastric reservoir, stomach prolapse around the band, gastric perforations, intractable vomiting, severe adhesive syndrome, among other complications, led to this approach being rapidly abandoned. Nevertheless, amid all these setbacks, one thing became clear from these experiences: silicone was the ideal material for constructing the band, as it produced virtually no adverse reactions in patients. With this knowledge, Austrian surgeon Gerhard Szinicz introduced the next crucial modification. Working in rabbits, he developed a circumferential silicone band containing an internal balloon connected to a subcutaneous port. The volume of the balloon and the size of the band could be adjusted by adding or removing saline through the port (Szinicz et al., 1989). Building on this idea, two groups of surgeons, almost simultaneously, began to work to apply this concept to humans.

In 1985, Dag Hallberg and Peter Forsell in Sweden described what would later become known as the Swedish Adjustable Gastric Band (SAGB) (Hallberg & Forsell, 1985). In parallel, Lubomyr Kuzmak, a Ukrainian surgeon working in the United States, reported the clinical use of an inflatable Silastic band that would later be known as the American Band or Lap-Band (Kuzmak, 1986). Both devices were connected to a subcutaneous port through which their size could be adjusted. The next major milestone came in 1995, when Belgian surgeon Mitiku Belachew first described the laparoscopic placement of an adjustable gastric band (Belachew et al., 1995). His article, which included a description of the technique, caused a sensation in the bariatric surgery community. The surgical procedure was relatively simple compared to other operations, the learning curve was short, and most importantly, it was reversible and did not alter the normal anatomy of the gastrointestinal tract.

That same year, the first world congress on adjustable gastric banding was held, where Belachew and many others presented their techniques and very preliminary but apparently promising results. At this point, both the Lap-Band and the SAGB were available in virtually every country except the United States. The combination of all these factors led to an unprecedented surge in the number of bariatric procedures performed. Physicians and patients alike became interested in and demanded the procedure. Similarly, public interest and media influence massively promoted the surgery (Steffen, 2008). FDA approval for the use of the Lap-Band in the United States in 2001 only further amplified this phenomenon.

Thus, gastric banding went from being an unknown procedure to accounting for 24.4% of bariatric surgeries in 2003. By 2008, it was the most commonly performed bariatric surgery worldwide, representing 42.3% of all obesity interventions (Angrisani et al., 2015). Countries such as Switzerland went from having only two hospitals performing bariatric surgery to more than 50 centers dedicated to obesity surgery, where adjustable gastric band placement was virtually the only procedure performed (Steffen, 2008).

However, the dream of having found the perfect surgery to end the obesity epidemic was short-lived. In 2010, reports began to emerge that contradicted the initially promising results. The percentage of weight loss achieved with the band was much lower than with other procedures and was not sustained over time. Once patients adapted, they regained most of the weight they had lost. Additionally, problems such as band migration or slippage often required removal due to intractable vomiting. As a result, revisional surgery for band removal, with or without conversion to another bariatric procedure, became routine in the same centers that for years had focused almost exclusively on band placement. Reports of up to 60% band removal appeared in the years following (Dargent, 2017). By 2013, gastric band placement accounted for only 10% of all bariatric surgeries (Angrisani et al., 2015). In 2016, the manufacturer announced the withdrawal of the SAGB from the market.

Beyond the undeniable problem of obesity, which warranted a vigorous and decisive response, the question arises as to how a surgical procedure that was virtually newly described, with unproven benefits and not fully understood implications, could so quickly become the most commonly performed obesity surgery worldwide. Was it the urgent need to do something in the face of the obesity pandemic? This seems unlikely, as there were already a number of available procedures, described long before the gastric band, with proven results and already in use. Could it be that the desire for the ideal, dream surgery blinded the surgical community? Again, this is improbable, as physicians are, above all, scientists trained to evaluate matters based on outcomes, and while some may have succumbed to this, it is almost impossible to believe that the entire surgical world would become blind to reality. So, what happened? The answer likely lies in the bandwagon effect, one of the cognitive biases that most strongly influences our everyday decisions.

Definition

The bandwagon effect is a cognitive bias in which individuals tend to adopt beliefs, behaviors, positions, or make decisions based on what the majority of people think, do or decide, without subjecting these to a critical analysis process and disregarding their own convictions or previous actions. Thus, as more people adopt a particular belief or behavior, many others are "swept along" to follow suit, regardless of what existing evidence or common sense may suggest. The fundamental idea behind this bias is that if many people do or think something, then this thought or behavior must be correct or appropriate for a given situation. While this idea may satisfy the need for belonging, provide a sense of security and even facilitate social integration, it can also lead to catastrophic errors.

In the previous example, when the laparoscopic adjustable gastric band was first described, it appeared to be the ideal procedure to address the problem of obesity: reversible, relatively simple and easy to learn, with no modifications to the anatomy of the gastrointestinal tract, and applicable to most patients. This novel idea, consistent with what was desired, seemingly beneficial and developed at the moment of greatest need, quickly gained followers. When its proponents began to present their successful results and organize scientific activities to disseminate their experiences, the impression was created that the entire surgical community was performing or should be performing the procedure, and that those who did not would be left behind or become obsolete. The lack of solid and stable scientific evidence or consideration of potential adverse consequences was overlooked. Thus, the insertion of the adjustable gastric band became the most commonly performed procedure for treating obesity in a very short period of time, as it was perceived as the thing to do. The consequences were disastrous.

History

The term bandwagon effect was adopted in psychology from the context of nineteenth-century American politics. A bandwagon (Fig. 16.1) was a type of musical wagon that carried a group or band during a parade, circus, or other entertainment event. In 1848, Dan Rice, the most famous clown of the era, invited then-presidential candidate Zachary Taylor to join his circus wagons as part of his campaign for the presidency of the United States. Rice used his enormous popularity to attract crowds to campaign events, and as Taylor's campaign became more successful and it was clear he would win, the phrase "*jump on the bandwagon*" became the way to attract all those who wanted to be associated (Carlyon, 2004). By 1900, bandwagons had become a regular feature of all American political campaigns, and the phrase "jump on the bandwagon" had evolved to refer to anyone wishing to associate themselves with success, regardless of whom they were aligning with.

Although this phenomenon has been known since that time, it was not fully understood until many years later, initially with the work of Muzafer Sherif on group processes and frames of reference in 1935 (Relations, University of Oklahoma. Institute of Group Relations & Sherif, 1961), and subsequently with Solomon Asch's studies on group conformity in the 1950s, which finally brought the concept into the field of psychology. In his famous line experiments, participants were asked to determine which of three presented lines matched a reference line in the presence of a majority group (7–9 people). The task was quite simple and unambiguous, as the design of the lines left no room for doubt. Before each individual announced their choice, the majority group (actors prepared for the occasion), deliberately and

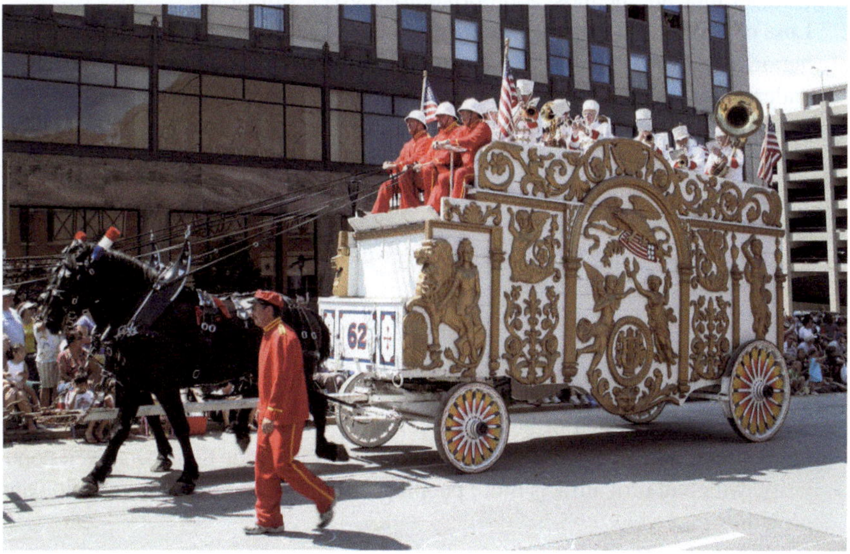

Fig. 16.1 Bandwagon (public domain). *Source* Freekee—Own work

unanimously gave an incorrect answer. The aim of the study was to assess how this behavior would influence the participant's choice (Asch, 1956). Despite the answer being incorrect, one third of the participants chose in accordance with the majority, which was an extraordinarily high number considering that in the control group (without the majority's opinion), 100% of participants gave the correct answer. To further emphasize the issue, after the experiment, participants were interviewed and the true purpose of the experiment was explained, along with questions about their mental process when choosing a line. The responses were even more striking, as virtually all the participants who answered incorrectly had felt that something was odd about the group's choice. However, they chose to abandon their initial opinion and go along with the majority. Multiple studies spanning most areas of human knowledge have confirmed these initial findings, expanding current understanding of this bias.

Impact

As previously mentioned, the consequences of the bandwagon effect extend to nearly all facets of life and human behavior. Among the most significant are:

At the Personal Level:

1. **Adoption or rejection of beliefs, attitudes, and behaviors:** Depending on what is perceived as most popular or common, individuals adopt or discard convictions or behaviors without subjecting them to critical analysis and without considering whether they are the most appropriate for a given situation.
2. **Loss of individual critical thinking:** By allowing decisions to be guided by the majority, personal analytical capacity and evaluation of one's own criteria are undermined, as they are set aside in favor of the apparent wisdom of the crowd.
3. **Modification of habits or lifestyles:** By adopting the behaviors of the majority, individuals change or acquire new habits in order to fit in or be part of the majority, abandoning those personal traits and characteristics that define authenticity.
4. **Emotional fragility:** By constantly depending on external validation from the masses as the defining measure of what is right or wrong in decisions and actions, self-confidence is weakened.

At the Collective Level:

1. **Expansion of political and social movements:** Once a political or social movement, whether justified or not, is perceived as the most common or as gaining momentum, many people will end up joining it solely due to its perceived popularity, which in turn attracts more people, creating a cascade of propagation and growth.

2. **Spread of false news and creation of opinion matrices:** Any information or opinion associated with the majority will be rapidly disseminated and accepted, regardless of its validity and/or relevance to a particular context.
3. **Social polarization:** By following the opinions of the apparent majority, relationships with people who share similar thoughts and behaviors become closer, while relationships with those holding different beliefs become more distant. This phenomenon within a society ultimately generates factions with completely opposing views on how the collective should behave or be governed, making it difficult to reach agreements, as both sides feel they are the majority and possess the absolute truth.

Examples in Medical and Surgical Practice

Medicine and surgery, as fundamentally human disciplines in constant pursuit of excellence, thrive on the ongoing exchange of ideas and experiences among colleagues through publications, conferences, or direct contact. Here, the consequences of the bandwagon effect are multiple, diverse, and inevitable. Among the most significant are:

1. **Premature adoption of surgical techniques and procedures,** such as the case of the adjustable gastric band, regardless of the existing evidence, simply because the majority are doing it and there is a desire not to be left behind or become obsolete.
2. **Unquestioning adherence to clinical practice guidelines,** created by majority consensus but not adapted to every particular situation or not developed on solid evidence, as occurs with rare diseases or novel scenarios. For example: ordering an abdominal CT scan for a patient presenting to the emergency department with abdominal pain, following the clinical practice guideline without noting clear signs of acute appendicitis.
3. **Inappropriate and excessive use of diagnostic tests,** disregarding proper clinical judgment or necessity, simply to comply with the apparent new standard of "excellence" and not be "left behind" by what is "new and trending." For example: ordering a PET-CT in the initial evaluation of every cancer patient, regardless of biological behavior, clinical stage, or the likelihood that the study will provide relevant information for patient management.
4. **Unnecessary prescription of new medications** heavily promoted by the industry and supposedly widely used by colleagues, but without clear benefits, simply to stay in line with "the latest trend." For example: abandoning rational antibiotic use in the management of acute cholecystitis to prescribe the latest quinolone released on the market, which is touted as a panacea for intra-abdominal infections.

5. **Perpetuation of inappropriate or unnecessary practices** simply because everyone does it, without questioning their validity or necessity, even in the face of evidence demonstrating their lack of effectiveness. For example: the use of drains after thyroidectomy or to monitor the duodenal stump after gastrectomy.

How to Avoid Falling into this Bias

1. **Foster critical thinking and reflective decision-making:** Regardless of who or how many people think or do a certain thing, always subject any new information or action to a careful and thorough analysis. Likewise, acquire tools that enable rigorous and impartial evaluation of any new scientific evidence that is presented.
2. **Be wary of any new idea that is adopted too quickly:** When faced with any new medication, procedure, or diagnostic study that is rapidly accepted and/or promoted, systematically reflect on why it has become so popular, whether there is truly evidence to support it, and whether it fits the particular situation and context of the patients.
3. **Be aware of the existence and influence of the bias:** Knowing and recognizing that the thoughts and actions of others influence one's own beliefs and decisions is an essential step to resist social pressure and make better decisions.
4. **Seek diverse opinions:** Always consider the widest possible range of assessments and perspectives, especially those that differ from the prevailing thought or behavior, in order to achieve a more balanced judgment and make better decisions. For this same purpose, in group meetings, assign in advance one or more people to deliberately defend the opposing view or opinion to that of the majority, regardless of the group's tendency or even their own position.
5. **Pay attention to cognitive dissonance:** Cognitive dissonance, defined as the psychological discomfort that unconsciously arises when individuals sense contradictions between their attitudes, beliefs, and behaviors, is an invaluable tool for avoiding this bias. Instead of silencing it or trying to explain and justify decisions and actions, learn to use it as a warning sign that something needs to be thought about more carefully.
6. **Slow down decision-making:** Before reaching any resolution, consider alternatives that go against the majority opinion, take time to reflect, thoroughly evaluate motivations, and avoid impulsive decisions.
7. **Develop self-esteem and confidence:** Strengthen personal confidence and security so as not to depend on the validation of the majority to feel valuable and successful.

References

Angrisani, L., Santonicola, A., Iovino, P., Formisano, G., Buchwald, H., & Scopinaro, N. (2015). Bariatric surgery worldwide 2013. *Obesity Surgery, 25*(10), 1822–1832. https://doi.org/10.1007/s11695-015-1657-z

Asch, S. E. (1956). Studies of independence and conformity: I. A minority of one against a unanimous majority. *American Psychological Association*. https://doi.org/10.1037/h0093718

Belachew, M., Legrand, M., Vincenti, V. V., Deffechereux, T., Jourdan, J. L., Monami, B., & Jacquet, N. (1995). Laparoscopic placement of adjustable silicone gastric band in the treatment of morbid obesity: How to do it. *Obesity Surgery, 5*(1), 66–70. https://doi.org/10.1381/096089295765558196

Carlyon, D. (2004). *Dan rice: The most famous man you've never heard of*. PublicAffairs. https://books.google.com.co/books?id=S_TTtAEACAAJ

Dargent, J. (2017). Laparoscopic gastric banding: Game over? *Obesity Surgery, 27*(8), 1914–1916. https://doi.org/10.1007/s11695-017-2710-x

Dumon, K. R., & Murayama, K. M. (2011). Bariatric surgery outcomes. *Surg Clin North Am, 91*(6), 1313–1338, x. https://doi.org/10.1016/j.suc.2011.08.014

Finkelstein, E. A., Fiebelkorn, I. C., & Wang, G. (2003). National medical spending attributable to overweight and obesity: How much, and who's paying? *Health Aff (Millwood), Suppl Web Exclusives*, W3–219–226. https://doi.org/10.1377/hlthaff.w3.219

Hallberg, D., & Forsell, P. (1985). Ballongband vid behandling av massive obesity. *Swedish Surgery, 43*(2), 106.

Hensrud, D. D., & Klein, S. (2006). Extreme obesity: A new medical crisis in the United States. *Mayo Clinic Proceedings, 81*(10 Suppl), S5-10. https://doi.org/10.1016/s0025-6196(11)61175-0

Kelly, T., Yang, W., Chen, C. S., Reynolds, K., & He, J. (2008). Global burden of obesity in 2005 and projections to 2030. *International Journal of Obesity, 32*(9), 1431–1437. https://doi.org/10.1038/ijo.2008.102

Kuzmak, L. (1986). Silicone gastric banding: A simple and effective operation for morbid obesity. *Contemporary Surgery, 28*, 13–18.

National Institutes of Health. (2001). Publications and reports of the surgeon general. In *The surgeon general's call to action to prevent and decrease overweight and Obesity*. Office of the Surgeon General (US).

Ogden, C. L., Carroll, M. D., Curtin, L. R., McDowell, M. A., Tabak, C. J., & Flegal, K. M. (2006). Prevalence of overweight and obesity in the United States, 1999–2004. *JAMA, 295*(13), 1549–1555. https://doi.org/10.1001/jama.295.13.1549

Powers, K. A., Rehrig, S. T., & Jones, D. B. (2007). Financial impact of obesity and bariatric surgery. *Medical Clinics of North America, 91*(3), 321–338, ix. https://doi.org/10.1016/j.mcna.2007.01.001

Relations, University of Oklahoma. Institute of Group Relations., & Sherif, M. (1961). *Intergroup conflict and cooperation: The Robbers Cave experiment* (Vol. 10). University Book Exchange Norman, OK.

Steffen, R. (2008). The history and role of gastric banding. *Surg Obes Relat Dis, 4*(3 Suppl), S7-13. https://doi.org/10.1016/j.soard.2008.04.002

Szinicz, G., Müller, L., Erhart, W., Roth, F. X., Pointner, R., & Glaser, K. (1989). Reversible gastric banding" in surgical treatment of morbid obesity–results of animal experiments. *Research in Experimental Medicine (Berl), 189*(1), 55–60. https://doi.org/10.1007/bf01856030

Wilkinson, L. H. (1980). Reduction of gastric reservoir capacity. *American Journal of Clinical Nutrition, 33*(2 Suppl), 515–517. https://doi.org/10.1093/ajcn/33.2.515

Wilkinson, L. H., & Peloso, O. A. (1981). Gastric (reservoir) reduction for morbid obesity. *Archives of Surgery, 116*(5), 602–605. https://doi.org/10.1001/archsurg.1981.01380170082014

References

Chapter 17
Reactive Devaluation. Ignaz Semmelweis and Handwashing

The Problem

By the 1830s, puerperal fever had become a major public health problem. Originally described by Hippocrates, without a specific name, for centuries it was attributed to an abnormal flow of lochia (Mingote & Nava, 2016). As a rare disease limited to the domain of midwives, who were responsible for childbirth without scientific or formal training, it attracted little interest from the medical community. For more than fifteen hundred years, Hippocrates' original causal explanation went unquestioned, not even when the disease acquired its name in 1716 (Strother, 1718). However, in the eighteenth century, with the gradual development of academic medicine and the industrial revolution, this situation began to change due to two fundamental events: first, the establishment of medical leaders, which turned childbirth into a medical act; and second, the creation and development of hospitals, which led to the emergence of maternity wards. This progress, however, also brought a change in the behavior of the disease. Case reports, which had been rare for centuries, began to increase exponentially. While it might be thought that this rise was due to childbirth now receiving more "*scientific*" attention, the increase in cases, which led to genuine epidemics, was seen only in hospitals, never when births were attended at home by midwives. By the first half of the nineteenth century, maternal deaths from puerperal fever had reached alarming levels. In London, between 1831 and 1843, maternal mortality was 10 per 10,000 for home births and 600 per 10,000 in the Lying Hospital. Similar figures were reported throughout Europe (Churchill, 1849).

This problem, now clearly a medical one, demanded new explanations. Such differences could not be supported by an abnormal flow of lochia. From the second half of the eighteenth century, new hypotheses began to emerge: contagion from concurrent patients, the putrid environment of hospitals, seasonal causes, and even the use of very tight corsets by pregnant women were among suggestions (Bridson, 1996). However, none of these explanations gained general acceptance. By the first half of the nineteenth century, although a few physicians in Scotland and the United

A. Sanabria and C. Betancourt, *Cognitive Biases in Surgical Practice*,
https://doi.org/10.1007/978-3-032-20377-9_17

States had pointed out that doctors might play a role in the genesis of the disease, the most widely accepted explanation was "*miasmas,*" suspended particles of matter that transmitted the disease as a kind of "*poisonous vapor*." As a result, most hospitals focused their efforts on improving ventilation in maternity wards (Lane et al., 2010).

Within all this chaos, one hospital had managed to remain unaffected by the problem. The Allgemeine Krankenhouse, General Hospital, in Vienna, with its policy of keeping childbirth in the hands of midwives with minimal medical involvement, had managed to keep the maternal mortality rate from puerperal fever below 1%. In 1824, however, this situation changed dramatically. The new head of the maternity service, Dr. Johann Klein, in line with practices in other European centers, decided to involve physicians and medical students in childbirth, who simultaneously began performing autopsies as part of the study of normal and pathological anatomy in women. These changes led to an increase in maternal mortality from puerperal fever, which rose to 7.5% (Salaverry García, 2013). Nevertheless, this increase went unnoticed, as it was similar to or lower than that seen in major European health centers. In 1834, to meet the growing demand for patients, a second maternity ward was created, in which care was also provided by physicians, students, and midwives. In 1839, for educational reasons (it was necessary to train both physicians and midwives, with quite different competencies and skills required for each profession), it was decided to reorganize the maternity services. Ward 1, dedicated to the training of physicians, was placed under care of students and doctors. Ward 2, intended for the training of midwives, remained under their responsibility, with minimal medical involvement, as had been the case until 1824. Soon, differences in puerperal fever mortality between the two wards became apparent. Between 1841 and 1846, mortality in Ward 1 ranged from 13 to 17%, reaching as high as 50% during an epidemic period. In contrast, in Ward 2, mortality was only 1.5% (Cwikel, 2008). These figures were alarming, as it was safer to give birth in the street than in Ward 1 of the Vienna Hospital. Moreover, considering that the Allgemeine Krankenhaus was at the time the most renowned European institution for medical study and research, the situation was utterly unacceptable. However, for the hospital authorities, the problem was not considered particularly significant. The differences were attributed to the fact that the doctors and students in Ward 1, all men, were rougher and sharper in attending deliveries than their counterparts in Ward 2, female midwives. All this changed, however, with the arrival of Dr. Ignaz Semmelweis in 1846.

Semmelweis (Fig. 17.1) was born in Hungary in 1818. After several turbulent years of study between Hungary and Austria, he graduated as a physician from the University of Vienna in 1844. As an outstanding student, he remained at the University and obtained a diploma as an obstetrics´ expert in 1846. That same year, he won the competition to become assistant to Dr. Klein and became head of Ward 1 of the maternity department at the Vienna General Hospital. Aware of the problem of maternal deaths from puerperal fever and the difference between the two wards, he decided to focus on finding the cause of this disparity. Methodically and systematically, he studied and ruled out the various hypotheses that had been proposed: climatic influences, overcrowding in the rooms, improper use of forceps, excessive roughness during vaginal examination and delivery, excessive anxiety due to the presence of a priest in the maternity ward, etc. When everything had been ruled out, an incident directed him in the right direction. In early 1847, Dr. Jakob Kolletschka, professor of pathology at the University and a close friend of Semmelweis, suffered a minor accidental cut on his hand while performing an autopsy on a woman who had died of puerperal fever. Days later, he died of "*pathologist's pyemia*" (Cwikel, 2008), a condition similar to puerperal fever, with the difference that the victim was a man who had never been pregnant. Moreover, as a pathologist, he was not part of the staff working in the maternity ward. This event led Semmelweis to focus on the additional activities performed by the students and doctors attending deliveries in Ward 1. He quickly noticed that they performed autopsies before beginning their obstetric duties and often moved from one activity to another wearing the same clothing. It was not uncommon to find remnants of necrotic and devitalized tissue on the clothes and hands of students and doctors. Based on these observations, Semmelweis formulated a hypothesis linking puerperal fever to "*cadaveric particles*" carried from the dead to laboring mothers by doctors and students. This explained both the cases of puerperal fever and the difference compared to Ward 2, where midwives did not perform autopsies. To test his theory, he introduced a mandatory measure in May 1847, even without Dr. Klein's authorization: all students and doctors, without exception, were required to wash their hands and scrub their nails with a sodium hypochlorite solution upon leaving the autopsy room and before entering the maternity ward to attend deliveries. Later, realizing that transmission could occur from one mother to another, he extended the rule to require handwashing between each patient. He meticulously studied and recorded the mortality rates after implementing the measure, and by the second half of 1847, mortality from puerperal fever had dropped to 3%, and by 1848 it was reduced to 1.2%. The difference in mortality between the two wards disappeared. Eager for his measure to be adopted throughout Europe, he published his results in 1848 and presented them at the Royal Medical and Surgical Society of Vienna in early 1849 (Cwikel, 2008). However, instead of being recognized for his discovery, his findings were met with deep rejection by the medical community. His discoveries implied that, in one way or another, physicians were responsible for the deaths, something never before considered and entirely contrary to the ethos of the medical profession. Although the evidence was solid, its implications were a clear affront to the establishment. When questioned about the definition of "*cadaveric particles*," he could not explain their origin (at the time, the existence of bacteria and microorganisms was unknown, knowledge that would come more than half a century later). His results were dismissed and labeled as non-reproducible and later as false, even by his own superior, Dr. Klein, who attributed the reduction in mortality to a new ventilation system installed at the time. By the second half of 1849, his contract was terminated and he had to leave the Vienna General Hospital. His successor, Dr. Braun, eliminated all the measures Semmelweis had implemented, following Klein's instructions. By 1850, maternal mortality from puerperal fever had returned to pre-1847 levels, and the difference between the two wards reappeared (Gillies, 2005).

Handwashing is now the main and most effective measure to reduce the transmission of hospital-acquired infections. The fact that its implementation was once

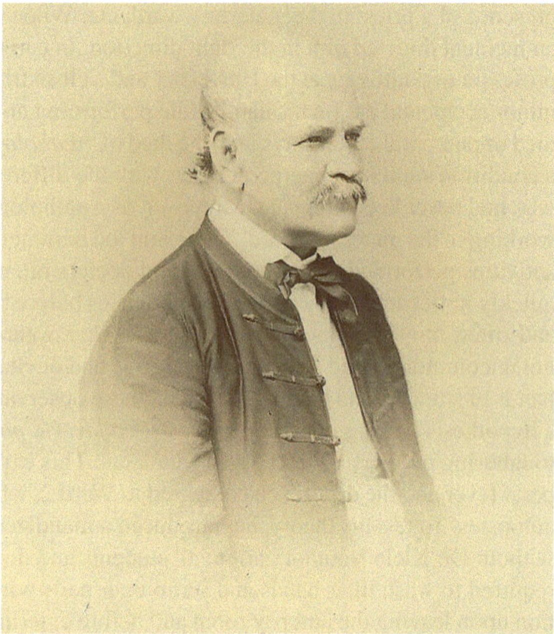

Fig. 17.1 Ignaz Semmelweis (public domain). *Source* József Borsos / Albert Doctor—Ágnes Szemerédi: A fényképészet úttörői, OSZK blog, 2022

rejected is both astonishing and extraordinary. However, the story of Semmelweis is tragically clear. The question that arises after 200 years is why a measure that was easy to implement and saved lives was rejected. Semmelweis had trained as a physician and obstetrician at the Vienna General Hospital and was not an unknown figure within the medical community of the Austrian capital, so his authority was recognized. Although statistics as a science did not yet exist, Semmelweis's numbers were robust enough to support his argument, and no sophisticated analysis was needed to understand the success of the measure. Moreover, maternal mortality, with all its familial and social repercussions, was a matter of great importance in the nineteenth-century Vienna. At the same time, germs were unknown at the time, and it was widely accepted that diseases were transmitted by "*miasmas*," so the lack of identification of a pathogenic agent seems more like a pretext for not accepting the evidence than a genuine reason. So, what happened? The answer likely lies in reactive devaluation, one of the cognitive biases that most hinders reaching agreements in negotiations and conflict resolution.

Definition

Reactive devaluation is the biased cognitive process by which the opinions, arguments, or proposals put forward by another party are undervalued and rejected, especially if that party is perceived as negative, antagonistic, or opposed to oneself.

This phenomenon distorts the perception of the true value of things, assigning less importance or relevance to ideas simply because they are presented by someone or something we consider to be contrary or to have interests different from our own. As with most cognitive biases, a difficult question, how important or true is the idea or proposal being presented? is replaced by an easier one, how close or aligned am I with the person presenting the idea or proposal? Negative answers will lead to the dismissal of the proposal, without giving it the proper space and time to assess its relevance or truthfulness.

In Semmelweis's case, his ideas indirectly held physicians responsible for maternal deaths, something that had never happened before and clearly ran counter to the aims of the profession. Although this was not his intention, his arguments quickly made him an antagonistic figure, opposed to the entire Viennese medical community. His proposals were not seen as coming from an obstetrician seeking to end puerperal fever, but from an "*enemy*" of physicians who blamed them for mothers' deaths. Reactive devaluation did the rest, with the results we already know. The "*Semmelweis effect*," a term coined from this story (Leary & Wilson, 1993) to describe the tendency to reject evidence that contradicts established beliefs or paradigms, is one of the many ways in which reactive devaluation can manifest.

History

Reactive devaluation as a cognitive bias was proposed by Lee Ross and Constance Stillinger in 1988 (Ross & Stillinger, 1991), based on a series of experiments they conducted beginning in 1986. In these experiments, at the end of the USSR and the Cold War, they asked American citizens for their opinion on a hypothetical plan for massive nuclear arms reduction in the United States and the Soviet Union. To the researchers' surprise, acceptance of the plan depended solely on the hypothetical origin of the proposal. If the proposal came from President Reagan (United States), acceptance of the disarmament program was 90%. If it came from a neutral party, it was 80%, but if it came from President Gorbachev (Soviet Union), only 44% of respondents accepted it. Multiple experiments have corroborated the existence and scope of reactive devaluation, establishing it as one of the main barriers to reaching agreements in any setting.

Impact

Humans are naturally social beings who depend on interaction with others for personal and collective development. The exchange of ideas and proposals, debate, and the ability to reach agreements are fundamental pillars for social progress. In this sense, it is not difficult to imagine the negative effects of reactive devaluation in limiting or diminishing our capacity for these processes. Among the most important are:

At the Personal Level:

1. **Reduced ability to resolve disputes and reach agreements:** Whether at work, at home with family, at a party with friends, or in the supermarket line, conflicts are inevitable and part of daily life. The ability to engage in dialogue, listen to the other party's opinion, and eventually reach an agreement is essential for a fulfilling life in society. Reactive devaluation diminishes this ability by systematically undermining the opinion and position of the other party involved.
2. **Subjective evaluation of others' opinions:** The ideas and concepts of those we interact with are necessary to construct the reality of the world around us, providing different perspectives and viewpoints on daily situations. These allow us to make better decisions. Reactive devaluation impairs this ability, introducing subjectivity into the analysis and devaluing other opinions, especially if they come from people with opposing views.
3. **Need for control:** Reactive devaluation leads to a desire to control those around us, especially those who are dependent. In this way, one may come to consider one's own opinion and perspective as the only real and important ones, systematically dismissing those of others and seeking to impose one's own.

At the Collective Level:

1. **Creation of stereotypes and prejudice:** By constantly discrediting and belittling the opinions of "*opposing*" individuals, generalization and stigmatization are promoted, leading to unjust exclusion and the creation of stereotypes within society. Once established, these stereotypes generate a vicious cycle of rejection, exclusion, and social division.
2. **Weakening of the social fabric:** When attitudes of discredit, disdain, distrust, and inability to reach agreements prevail, social bonds and connections are weakened, hindering the development of collaborative and enriching relationships by depriving us of the trust, respect, and solidarity necessary for their establishment. Thus, social organization, essential for our collective functioning, is undermined, resulting in tensions, conflicts, and eventual division within society.

Examples in Medical and Surgical Practice

Medical practice, with its complexity and specialization, makes teamwork necessary and indispensable. For this to be effective, the exchange of opinions and the establishment of agreements are fundamental. In this complex and challenging environment, reactive devaluation affects all facets of medical practice. Among the most important are:

1. **Rejection of colleagues' opinions** which may represent important perspectives for accurate diagnosis, treatment, and prognosis, especially in difficult cases or situations. For example, rejecting a colleague's appropriate surgical approach proposed during a departmental meeting simply because there was a disagreement over another patient in a previous meeting, where opposing viewpoints were presented.
2. **Inability to reach agreements** that would allow for better diagnostic or treatment options for a given patient. For example, deciding to operate on a patient with borderline resectable cancer because the oncologist was unwilling to consider the neoadjuvant alternative due to previous disagreements.
3. **Isolationism.** When agreements cannot be reached, medical practice can become an isolated exercise, lacking the healthy and necessary interaction among colleagues that leads to more accurate decisions regarding diagnosis, treatment, and prognosis. For example, ceasing to attend departmental case discussions because "they *never say or conclude anything relevant.*"
4. **Formation of factions.** The formation of factions among individuals who do or do not share a particular opinion and/or perspective is reinforced by reactive devaluation, making it difficult to reach agreements that would improve patient care. Added is the time wasted in fruitless debates where each side only seeks to prove its point. For example, endless discussions in departmental meetings between *"interventionists"* and *"conservatives"* where each side defends its viewpoint without considering the relevance of the opposing arguments.

How to Avoid Falling into this Bias

1. **Recognize and accept the existence of reactive devaluation:** As with most biases, acknowledging its existence and learning how it affects our thinking is a necessary first step to overcoming it. In the case of reactive devaluation, this becomes even more important, as it directly influences how we judge others' ideas and proposals and any initiative presented to overcome it may end up being rejected.
2. **Recognize motivations:** When presenting arguments, and especially when making proposals, clearly state the reasons and interests behind them. This prevents the other party from assuming there are hidden, potentially harmful motives and facilitate acceptance of the proposal or idea.
3. **Specify the benefits for the other party:** When presenting proposals, clearly indicate how they align with the interests of the other party and the benefits of accepting them.
4. **Pause and reflect:** Whenever a new idea or proposal arises, train yourself to pause and reflect on the extent to which the person presenting it may influence your evaluation. Once this is determined, proceed to assess the proposal itself. By actively considering the potential effect of reactive devaluation, its impact can be mitigated.

5. **Involve mediators:** When proposals come from a neutral party rather than an opponent, reactive devaluation is reduced. In this regard, use debate moderators in meetings and employ intermediaries to present proposals to individuals with markedly different viewpoints. The presence of neutral third parties reduce the effect of reactive devaluation and allows for a more rational and objective evaluation of the proposals.

References

Bridson, E. (1996). Iatrogenic epidemics of puerperal fever in the 18th and 19th centuries. *British Journal of Biomedical Science, 53*(2), 134–139.

Churchill, F. (1849). *Essays on the puerperal fever and other diseases peculiar to women: Selected from the writings of British authors previous to the close of the eighteenth century* (Vol. 1). Sydenham Society.

Cwikel, J. (2008). Lessons from Semmelweis: A social epidemiologic update on safe motherhood. *Social Medicine, 3*(1), 19–35.

Gillies, D. (2005). Hempelian and Kuhnian approaches in the philosophy of medicine: The Semmelweis case. *Studies in History and Philosophy of Biological and Biomedical Sciences, 36*(1), 159–181. https://doi.org/10.1016/j.shpsc.2004.12.003

Lane, H. J., Blum, N., & Fee, E. (2010). Oliver Wendell Holmes (1809–1894) and Ignaz Philipp Semmelweis (1818–1865): Preventing the transmission of puerperal fever. *American Journal of Public Health, 100*(6), 1008–1009. https://doi.org/10.2105/ajph.2009.185363

Leary, T., & Wilson, R. A. (1993). *The game of life.* New Falcon Publications. https://books.google.com.co/books?id=TM4RAAAACAAJ

Mingote, L. S., & Nava, M. D. L. (2016). *Hippocratic Treatises IV*. Gredos. https://books.google.com.co/books?id=CpDODwAAQBAJ

Ross, L., & Stillinger, C. (1991). *Barriers to conflict resolution.* Blackwell Publishing. https://doi.org/10.1111/j.1571-9979.1991.tb00634.x

Salaverry García, O. (2013). Institutional iatrogenesis and maternal death. Semmelweis and puerperal fever. *Revista Peruana de Medicina Experimental y Salud Publica, 30*, 512–517. http://www.scielo.org.pe/scielo.php?script=sci_arttext&pid=S1726-46342013000300023&nrm=iso

Strother, E. (1718). *Criticon Febrium, or, a critical essay on fevers: With the Diagnosticks and methods of cure, in all the different species of them, to which is Prefix'd a large introduction concerning the use and abuse of the Mathematicks in Physick, and the basis on which indications are founded, where Also the Euodia Medicorum is Annex'd*. Charles Rivington.

Chapter 18
Authority Bias. The Queen's Anesthesia

The Problem

On October 16, 1846, William Thomas Green Morton, a dentist by profession, would forever change the surgical practice. That day, in a surgical amphitheater at Massachusetts General Hospital, the first pain-free surgery in history was performed following the anesthetic inhalation of ether vapors. Gilbert Abbott, just 20 years old, presented with a neck mass and was scheduled for resection by the renowned surgeon John Collins Warren, chief of surgery at the prestigious hospital (Fenster, 2001). After the usual surgical preparation, which included tying the patient to the operating table to keep him completely immobile, Abbott inhaled vapors from a glass globe containing a sponge soaked in ether provided by Morton. After a brief period of excitement, the patient fell into deep sleep. From that point, and for the next 10 min, Warren removed the tumor, with Abbott apparently unconscious throughout the entire procedure. A few minutes later, upon regaining consciousness, he was questioned by Warren about what he had felt and whether he remembered the surgery. To everyone's astonishment, the patient remembered nothing and only felt "*as if my neck had been scratched*" (Warren, 1848). The implications of Morton's discovery were extraordinary, almost magical. To operate on a patient calmly and precisely, without blood bursting in all directions and without the agonizing screams of pain, was the long-held dream of every surgeon. Since the beginnings of surgery, various strategies had been devised to immobilize patients, and nearly all surgeons had harrowing experiences with patients who had fled the operating rooms in a desperate attempt to escape pain, only to die later from uncontrollable bleeding. Surgical amphitheaters were not suitable for the general public, as many people could not withstand the combination of pain and blood presented there. For good reason, speed was the most prized attribute in a surgeon. All of this would change forever with Morton's discovery. Precision surgery, by anatomical planes, with minimal and rapidly controlled bleeding, would become a reality. Pain, with all its distressing consequences, would no longer be part of the surgical act. Not surprisingly, the 1846 article announcing Morton's anesthetic

A. Sanabria and C. Betancourt, *Cognitive Biases in Surgical Practice*,
https://doi.org/10.1007/978-3-032-20377-9_18

demonstration to the world is considered the most influential article ever published in the *New England Journal of Medicine* (Buckley, 2012). Less than a year later, surgeries under ether anesthesia were being performed virtually worldwide. However, contrary to what might be expected from such an extraordinary advance, many physicians in the United States and elsewhere remained skeptical, and anesthesia was still far from being a routine part of every surgical procedure. The constant positive testimonies from patients anesthetized with ether and the approval for its use by the American government were not enough to fully convince doctors and patients to adopt the practice. Concerns about the safety of the substances used, religious beliefs, supposed benefits of pain, alleged disadvantages of sedation, ego, and professional jealousy all combined to slow the global spread of a discovery that was clearly revolutionizing surgical practice (Meyer & Desai, 2015). In Europe, especially in England, opposition to the widespread use of anesthetics was particularly strong. There, many renowned surgeons openly opposed their use, considering them dangerous and unnecessary, "*an American hoax,*" which only benefited less skilled surgeons who could not perform surgeries quickly (vande Laar, 2024). All of this would change, however, in 1853 when Queen Victoria experienced the use of anesthesia during the birth of her eighth child.

Victoria of Hanover (Fig. 18.1) had ascended to the throne of the United Kingdom on June 20, 1837, following the death of her uncle William IV, who had left no surviving heirs. Daughter of Prince Edward, Duke of Kent, her grandfather was George III. By that time, the United Kingdom was already an established constitutional monarchy, where kings and queens theoretically held little direct political power. Despite this, during her 64-year reign, she would become a national and global icon, embodying the model of progress and strict values that would later be known as the Victorian era. During this period, the British Empire reached its greatest extent and development, becoming the world's leading power. Domestically, profound political and social reforms took place, such as the expansion of voting rights to the majority of the population and the establishment of "*Victorian morality*", a comprehensive set of values and ethical and behavioral norms that governed all aspects of social life, characterized by low tolerance for crime, a strict social code of conduct, and strong sexual repression (Bedarida, 1979). However, despite all her public successes and achievements, her personal and family life was far less satisfying. Married to her cousin Albert of Saxe-Coburg in 1840, by 1853, keeping in with the values of the era, she had already borne seven children. Contrary to what was publicized to the outside world, each of these had been a terrible experience. The Queen was unable to endure the excruciating pain of childbirth, which she referred to as an "*animal experience*" (vande Laar, 2024). Although all seven deliveries had proceeded without complications for her or the children, each had left a deep trauma in the Queen. Despite her strong character and iron determination, after each birth she fell into a deep depression, from which she recovered only to face another pregnancy. The problems extended to her relationship with her husband, and frequent arguments began to threaten its stability. By 1853, with the Queen pregnant for the eighth time and the prospect of another scary delivery, the situation was quite difficult. Concerned about what might happen, Prince Albert decided to try something different. Having heard

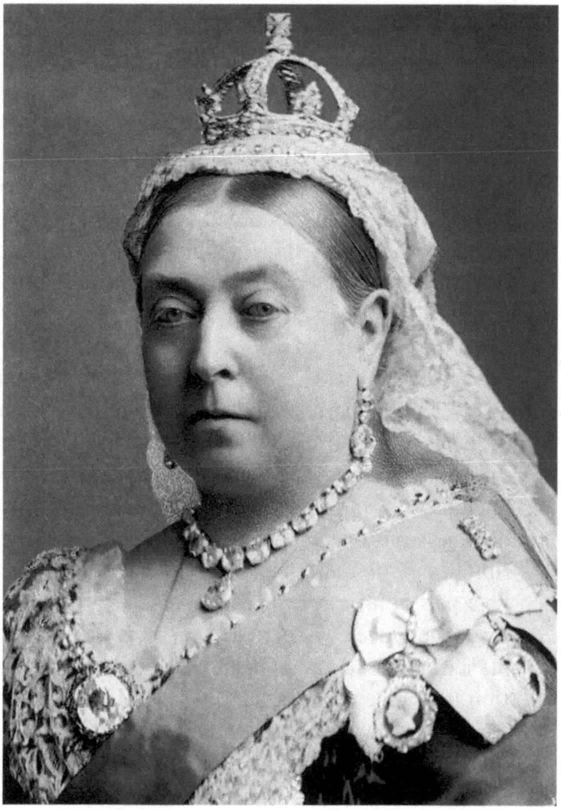

Fig. 18.1 Victoria of Hanover (public domain). *Source* Alexander Bassano—**Original text**: « *Scanned from the book 'The National Portrait Gallery History of the Kings and Queens of England' by David Williamson, ISBN 1,855,142,287, p. 153.*»

of the supposed benefits of anesthesia, he decided to contact John Snow to assist his wife during her next labor.

Snow (Fig. 18.2) was born in York in 1813. The son of a farmer, with no ties or connections to royalty or the political figures of the time, his beginnings were quite difficult. Nevertheless, through much sacrifice and dedication, he earned his degree as a physician and surgeon in 1844. Learning of the use of ether for the first time in England in December 1846 and then of chloroform in 1847, he devoted himself to extensively studying the use of both substances as anesthetic agents. His numerous experiences, initially in animals and later in humans, as well as the development of a series of instruments for the safe administration of these substances, had made him by 1853 the most famous anesthesiologist in London. His career, however, was not unlike that of every other physician dedicated to this art. Despite the many benefits of anesthesia, his practice as an anesthesiologist had yet to truly take off (Ramsay, 2006). Thus, the invitation to assist in the delivery of the most powerful woman in the world came as a huge surprise. John Snow, however, did not miss the opportunity. Armed with his instruments and chloroform, he presented himself at Buckingham Palace on April 7, 1853, to provide anesthesia to the Queen during the birth of her eighth child, Prince Leopold. Accompanied by Dr. James Clark, the royal obstetrician responsible for the delivery, he gradually administered 15 drops of chloroform to the Queen, at which point she confirmed that she no longer felt pain. To everyone's relief, the contractions remained just as strong. Fifty-three minutes later, at 1:13 am, the birth took place, with the placenta delivered without complications a few minutes later. The experience was a complete success. Snow, who meticulously recorded everything, later reported that the Queen had not experienced pain at any time and had always remained conscious and cooperative. Dr. Clark, who had attended the Queen in previous deliveries, confirmed Snow's report. The Queen herself later described it as *"the blessed chloroform, soothing and delightful beyond measure"* (vande Laar, 2024). The impact of the news was immediate. Despite criticism from some medical journals and condemnation from certain biblical scholars who believed that childbirth should be painful as stated in the Bible, the news spread rapidly around the world. In Europe, regardless of physicians' opinions, patients began to demand the use of anesthesia in all surgical procedures and in childbirth. In France, in particular, chloroform anesthesia became extremely popular and would be known as "*the Queen's anesthesia*" (vande Laar, 2024).

Without a doubt, anesthesia would eventually have become a routine and indispensable part of all surgical procedures, as its benefits were too great to be ignored. However, the Queen's experience served as a catalyst that undoubtedly enabled its acceptance and dissemination, allowing it to spread more quickly and efficiently. The question that arises more than 170 years later is why a single experience could so drastically eliminate the opinions and views that opposed the widespread use of anesthesia. Did these drugs become safe overnight? Clearly not. On the contrary, as their use increased, more reports of adverse events and even fatal outcomes emerged. Had the religious considerations based on what the Bible said about pain disappeared? Not at all. Did the rivalries, differences, and professional jealousies that existed among colleagues disappear because the Queen decided to receive anesthesia? No. So what happened? How can we explain the impact of the Queen's experience? The answer lies in the authority bias, one of the most common biases in everyday life.

Definition

Authority bias refers to the psychological tendency to accept the opinions, views, proposals, recommendations, and actions of individuals in positions of authority, power, and/or prominence (not necessarily experts) without subjecting them to a critical evaluation of their validity and/or accuracy. In this way, individuals are more easily influenced by the opinions of such people, as their viewpoints are considered more accurate and are rarely questioned or scrutinized. While hierarchical organization is fundamental to human development in society, both globally (countries) and individually (families, companies), by providing a structure that allows each person to occupy a more or less important role within the functioning of the collective, the unquestioning acceptance of the opinions or actions of those in the highest positions

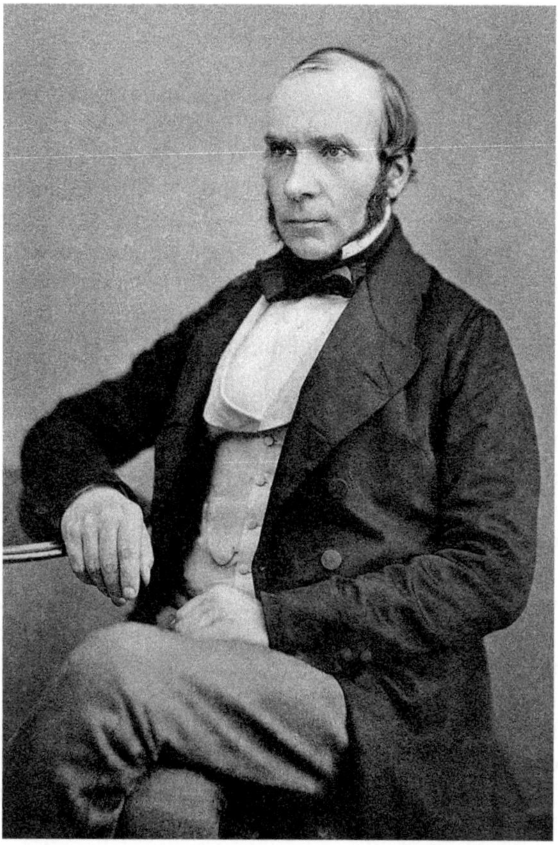

Fig. 18.2 John Snow (public domain). *Source* Wellcome trust corporate archive. Portrait of John Snow (1813–1858)

of power and/or authority can have catastrophic consequences, especially in today's world, where such positions are often not held by the most qualified and capable individuals, but rather by the most popular.

Within all the controversy surrounding the routine and widespread use of anesthesia, the Queen, for her own peculiar and particular reasons, decided to undergo chloroform administration. The experience involved what was, without a doubt, the most powerful and influential woman in the world. The Queen, however, was not an expert in anesthetics and probably was unaware of the ongoing debate in the medical community regarding their use. Nevertheless, once her positive experience became known, any doubts that might have existed about its use, especially among people who lacked clear knowledge of its advantages and disadvantages, quickly vanished. If the Queen was willing to use anesthesia, it would have to be good and even necessary. The most influential woman in the world would not subject herself to something that could endanger her life or safety. Therefore, there were no longer any doubts: anesthesia had to be useful, good, and necessary. The rest is history.

History

The term "*authority bias*" was introduced into the field of psychology following the work and publications of Stanley Milgram (Milgram, 1963). Milgram, an American psychologist of Jewish descent, was deeply affected by the events of the Holocaust and the contemporaneous trial in Israel of the Nazi war criminal Adolf Eichmann. He designed a series of experiments to try to understand why Nazi officers had been able to conduct orders from their superiors despite their tragic consequences. Were they simply following orders regardless of what those orders entailed, as Eichmann claimed in his defense? Or were they unscrupulous individuals as guilty as their superiors? How far could obedience go, regardless of what the orders suggested? Milgram designed multiple variations of a central experiment (Milgram, 1963). In this, individuals were recruited to function as "*teachers*" in an apparent study on learning and memory. The task was quite simple: as "*teachers*," they were to teach a "*learner*" a series of two-word associations. The teaching method, however, was unusual. Separated by a glass wall, the learner (who was an actor) sat in a kind of electric chair, where each mistake would be punished with an increasing electric shock, starting at 45 V and potentially reaching 450 V. The supposed electric shocks were fake, but everything was arranged so that the "*teacher*" believed they were real. Accompanying the "*teacher*" was the experimenter, who, in addition to supervising the experiment, made three things clear before starting: First, the electric shocks would be administered exclusively by the teacher; no one else had the authority or ability to do so. Second, everything was being recorded, so the "*teacher*" could not evade responsibility. Third, although the chair could deliver up to 450 V, shocks above 300 V could cause central nervous system disorders and even death. Milgram and his team assumed that the teachers would refuse to continue administering shocks, so they designed four phrases to be delivered sequentially by the experimenter to try to induce the "*teacher*" to continue with the experiment. If, after the fourth prompt, the teacher still refused, the experiment would end. Meanwhile, the actor playing the learner had been instructed to accompany each increasing shock with progressively greater displays of pain and suffering. Above 300 V, he should even begin to beg for his life. Milgram and his team had assumed that no one would be willing to administer shocks above 130 V. However, the results surprised the entire scientific community of the time. Sixty-five percent of participants administered shocks of 450 V (lethal in any scenario, if real), and no one stopped before 300 V (at which point there was a risk of death), regardless of the screams and obvious signs of pain from the learners. In response to apparent authority, human beings are capable of deeply disturbing actions. Numerous subsequent studies, with varying degrees of drama, have replicated Milgram's initial findings. In seeking an explanation, Milgram (Milgram, 2009) noted that when obeying authority, the individual feels like nothing more than an instrument executing the wishes of another person, and as such, is free from any responsibility; and Solomon Asch (Asch, 1951) showed that when a person lacks the ability or experience to make a decision, tends to follow that of the group or the group leader (authority figure) to which they belong.

Impact

Human beings function constantly and inevitably within hierarchical structures. Therefore, it is expected that the negative consequences of authority bias extend to all aspects of life. Among the most significant are:

At the Personal Level:

1. **Unquestioning acceptance of opinions and recommendations.**
2. **Blind obedience:** By accepting the views of authority figures without question, individuals tend to follow their recommendations and actions without assessing their appropriateness or relevance.
3. **Reduced evaluative capacity:** Similarly, by not questioning the opinions of those in positions of authority or power, the ability for critical analysis and evaluation is systematically diminished, making individuals more vulnerable to those opinions, as the brain forms the image and/or concept that "*if this person says it, it must be true or good.*"
4. **Inaccurate risk assessment:** By blindly trusting the opinion of authority figures, the ability to assess risk becomes distorted. Thus, their recommendations are considered safe or low risk, while their aversions are seen as dangerous and to be avoided. This is problematic, as even if the authority figure's opinion is correct, the specific situation from which the opinion is given does not necessarily reflect the context of the person receiving the recommendation and, therefore, may be inapplicable.

At the Collective Level:

1. **Expert power:** Authority bias exerts a profound effect on who is heard within any social group, organization, company, country, etc. Individuals in positions of authority within an organization are listened to more readily and even obligatorily, regardless of whether the person is an expert on the subject at hand. This phenomenon, known as " *expert power*," influences the proper dissemination of information and the decision-making process by magnifying the reach of the opinions of those in authority and limiting that of those with little or no authority, regardless of their knowledge or expertise on the subject.
2. **Creation of opinion chambers:** Due to their wider dissemination, the opinions of authority figures, whether correct or incorrect, easily create opinion chambers, as they are repeated and accepted by the population without consideration of their truthfulness or accuracy.
3. **Groupthink:** Authority bias also contributes to the formation of group thinking, especially in groups with highly authoritarian leaders. In such groups, to maintain harmony and cohesion, individuals accept the opinions of leaders or those with higher status within the group, setting aside the critical thinking and analysis necessary for sound decision-making.

Examples in Medical and Surgical Practice

The practice of medicine and surgery is hierarchical, with clearly defined roles and positions of authority established from the beginning of medical training and becoming more pronounced as training progresses. Thus, it is expected that the effects of authority bias are widespread. Among the most important examples are:

1. **Acquisition and transmission of behaviors and/or strategies for diagnosis, treatment, and follow-up:** In work groups or academic training programs, behaviors (protocols) are often established based on the opinions or committees of experts, which, once implemented, must be followed obligatorily by all group members, regardless of how long they have been in place or any new evidence that may have emerged. In turn, these "*protocols*" are passed on to each new generation entering the work group, with no room for discussion or dissent because "*this is how things are done here.*" For example, ordering a contrast-enhanced abdominal CT scan for every patient presenting with abdominal pain in the emergency department simply because it is mandated by the institution's management protocol.
2. **Unquestioning acceptance of opinions and recommendations:** In work groups, the opinion of the person with the most authority or experience is often regarded as absolute truth, without considering its validity, accuracy, or relevance, and systematically dismissing any evidence that may contradict it. For example, recommending laparoscopic repair of an inguinal hernia solely because it was suggested by the senior resident or department chief, who has neither evaluated nor is familiar with the patient.
3. **Rejection of opinions and recommendations:** The opinions of those with less authority are not heard or tend to be dismissed as lacking value. For example, disregard the opinion on physical examination findings during the initial assessment of a polytrauma patient by a first-year resident, even when relevant, because "*what could this new resident possibly know.*"
4. **Abandonment of independent judgment:** Being permanently subject to authority, physicians may become excessively dependent on it, neglecting their own judgment and confidence in their ability to make decisions in patient management. For example, the first-year resident who constantly consults the senior resident during the shift, even for the most basic matters, out of fear of "*making a mistake.*"

How to Avoid Falling into This Bias

1. **Separate the message from the messenger:** The most important step in avoiding this bias is to learn to focus on the content of the message, regardless of the position, role, or status of the person delivering it. Whenever possible, avoid knowing the source of the information before forming an opinion about it.

2. **Take time to think independently:** Before following any recommendation or adopting a particular position, logically consider what one would think or how one would behave if the suggestion had not been made. Then, compare this with the recommendation and decide, based on arguments, whether to accept or reject it.
3. **Cultivate critical thinking:** Systematically question all information received, regardless of its source. Develop a thought process that allows for the evaluation of opinions and recommendations, and subject all information to this process, no matter where it comes from.
4. **Actively search for other opinions:** Whenever a position must be taken or a decision made, search for as many opinions as possible from individuals with different experiences, backgrounds, and perspectives, considering all equally regardless of the position or role of the person expressing the opinion.
5. **Promote diversity of opinion:** Foster an environment in which everyone, regardless of their position or role, feels free to express their views or stance, encouraging open dialogue and constructive dissent at both the individual and collective levels. At the same time, promote a culture of continuous learning, in which authority figures can be readily challenged based on who has the most appropriate and up-to-date knowledge to address the various situations that may arise.
6. **Encourage evidence-based decision-making:** Promote a rational decision-making environment based on empirical evidence rather than the opinions of the most prominent figures within a group.

References

Asch, S. E. (1951). Effects of group pressure upon the modification and distortion of judgments. In *Groups, leadership and men; research in human relations* (pp. 177–190). Carnegie Press.

Bedarida, F. (1979). *A social history of England 1851–1990*. Methuen. https://books.google.com.co/books?id=l8XetwEACAAJ

Buckley, K. (2012, 7/10/2025). The most important article in NEJM history. *NEJM Journal Watch*. https://www.asahq.org/about-asa/newsroom/asa-in-the-news/2012/11/the-most-important-article-in-nejm-history

Fenster, J. M. (2001). *Ether day: The strange tale of America's greatest medical discovery and the haunted men who made it* (1st ed.). HarperCollins.

Meyer, R., & Desai, S. P. (2015). Accepting pain over comfort: Resistance to the use of anesthesia in the Mid-19th century. *Journal of Anesthesia History, 1*(4), 115–121. https://doi.org/10.1016/j.janh.2015.07.027

Milgram, S. (1963). Behavioral study of obedience. *Journal of Abnormal Psychology, 67*, 371–378. https://doi.org/10.1037/h0040525

Milgram, S. (2009). *Obedience to authority: An experimental view*. HarperCollins. https://books.google.com.co/books?id=vYGA45EODOgC

Ramsay, M. A. (2006). John Snow, MD: Anaesthetist to the queen of England and pioneer epidemiologist. *Proc (Bayl Univ Med Cent), 19*(1), 24–28. https://doi.org/10.1080/08998280.2006.11928120

vande Laar, A. (2024). *Under the knife: A history of surgery in 28 remarkable Operations*. St. Martin's Press. https://books.google.com.co/books?id=pJVJDwAAQBAJ

Warren, J. (1848). *Etherization: With surgical remarks.* Ticknor. https://collections.nlm.nih.gov/bookviewer?PID=nlm:nlmuid-66950810R-bk

Chapter 19
Outcome Bias. The Shead vs Hooley Case

The Problem

Surgical complications are adverse outcomes that may arise during or after surgery, negatively affecting the result of the procedure and the patient's prognosis. From the surgeon's perspective, they are a complex, unpleasant, and sensitive issue that entails enormous professional, moral, and ethical responsibility toward the patient, requiring the healthcare professional to constantly attempt to minimize their occurrence, prepare to diagnose them early and treat them promptly. From the patient's perspective, they are always a calamity that disrupts expectations regarding the benefits of surgery and may completely undermine the hope for resolution and cure of the disease that motivated the procedure. From the healthcare system's perspective, they represent increased hospital stays and resource expenditure and, in turn, serve as an indicator for evaluating the individual and collective performance of surgical services as well as the safety and quality of care.

Complications are also an inevitable part of every surgeon's professional career, as they are impossible to avoid, being associated with unpredictable circumstances that occur during surgery, with hidden patient conditions, with disease characteristics that cannot be improved or with unknown genetic factors. Thus, every surgeon's effort must be directed at keeping them to the lowest possible level, while at the same time accepting that, inevitably, they will have to deal with them. In these situations, it is valid to ask to what extent a surgeon should be held responsible for complication and, in the context of judicialization of medical practice, whether a surgeon should be considered at fault for a complication and punished accordingly. Recognizing that there are countless possibilities that can sway opinions in either direction, there is an increasing body of case law about medical civil liability (Fig. 19.1). Among these, few are more controversial than the Shead vs Hooley case, which occurred in the Australian state of New South Wales in the early twenty-first century.

In the late 1990s, Dr. Shead, a general surgery professor, performed a distal gastrectomy (antrectomy) plus vagotomy on Mrs. Hooley, who had previously

A. Sanabria and C. Betancourt, *Cognitive Biases in Surgical Practice*,
https://doi.org/10.1007/978-3-032-20377-9_19

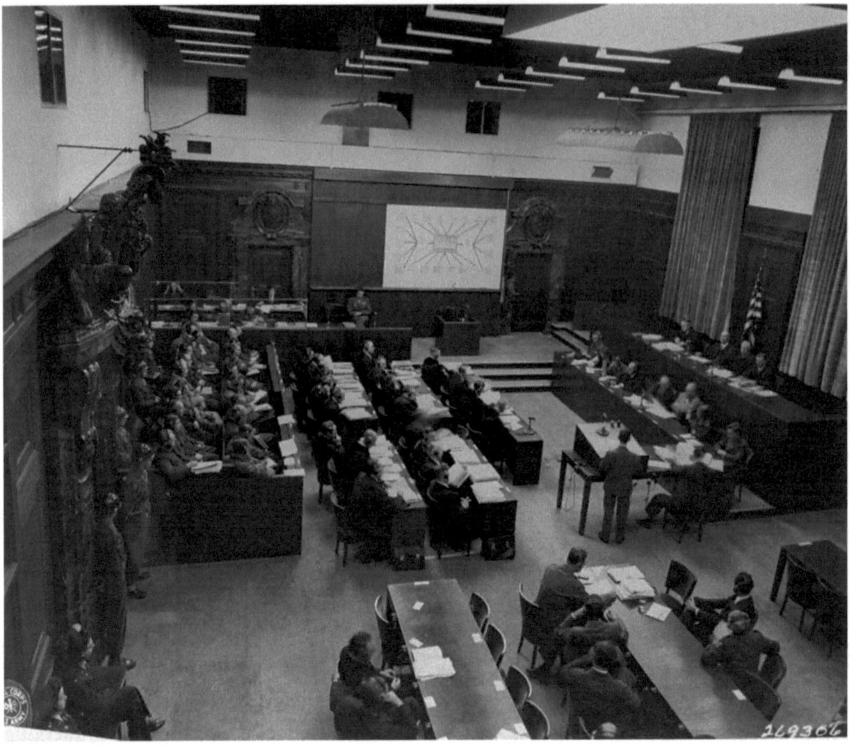

Fig. 19.1 Medical Judgments (public domain). Author unknown

consulted him for abdominal pain and persistent vomiting secondary to a chronic duodenal ulcer previously identified in several endoscopies. At the time, treatment with gastric acid secretion inhibitors was just beginning, and the surgical procedure was the treatment of choice for this disease. The surgery was a complete success and the duodenal ulcer healed. However, the patient's symptoms persisted. After several evaluations by various surgeons and gastroenterologists, Mrs. Hooley was diagnosed with gastroparesis (decreased or absent gastric motility), a complication rarely associated with vagotomy (1:10,000 patients undergoing the procedure) and which, in general, is treated with antrectomy, as was performed in this patient. Despite the confusing situation, Mrs. Hooley, following the recommendations of her gastroenterologist, Dr. Vickers, decided to undergo a total gastrectomy, which was duly performed by another surgeon, not Professor Shead. Although this new surgery was also successful and the patient's symptoms finally disappeared, the nutritional consequences of the new procedure left Mrs. Hooley completely incapacitated, and she was never able to work or conduct her usual activities again. Upset by the outcome of her initial surgery, the patient decided to sue Professor Shead for medical negligence (Hugh & Dekker, 2009).

During the trial, the prosecutor did not present any surgical evidence or argument, building the case around the fact that Mrs. Hooley had not been warned about the possibility of gastroparesis. Two expert surgeons brought in by the defense argued and presented solid evidence demonstrating that the surgery indicated by Professor Shead was the treatment of choice for the patient's disease; that antrectomy performed during the procedure was the solution commonly used for gastroparesis and, in this sense, warnings about this complication were unnecessary, since the procedure already included the potential cure for this rare complication, should it occur. In contrast, Dr. Vickers, the patient's gastroenterologist, who had recommended total gastrectomy with its disastrous consequences, presented evidence (later described as extravagant and unsatisfactory) to argue that the surgery performed by Professor Shead should not have been conducted. After all arguments were presented, the judge ruled in favor of Mrs. Hooley, finding the physician guilty of medical negligence. As a penalty, Professor Shead was ordered to compensate the patient with $933,363 for damages (Hugh & Dekker, 2009).

The verdict was appealed by Dr. Shead. The Court of Appeals was extremely critical of the evidence presented by Dr. Vickers, deciding that these arguments should be rejected and excluded from the case analysis. In response, Mrs. Hooley's lawyers presented Dr. Ellard, another gastroenterologist, who cited a series of articles indicating that the frequency of "delayed gastric emptying" after antrectomy with vagotomy was 3–9%. However, the same studies noted that all such problems were due to early obstructions of the gastroenteral anastomosis (usually from edema), which could be documented by endoscopy (something never performed on Mrs. Hooley) and typically resolved spontaneously. Gastroparesis, as such, was an almost non-existent problem. Despite all this information, which should have exonerated Professor Shead, the Court of Appeals decided to uphold the previous ruling, again finding the surgeon guilty of medical negligence and maintaining the penalty as established by the lower court (Hugh & Dekker, 2009).

Beyond the various legal aspects, processes, and repercussions—which are outside the scope of this text and fall entirely within the domain of legal professionals—it is impossible not to wonder how Professor Shead could have been found guilty. The surgery performed was a complete success, as evidenced by the resolution of the duodenal ulcer that had prompted it. Gastroparesis is an almost anecdotal complication of the procedure, and its potential treatment had already been included in the initial operation. The deterioration in the patient's quality of life was due to the total gastrectomy, not the initial surgery. It could even be argued, based on the articles presented to the Court of Appeals, that Mrs. Hooley rushed into the second surgery and that, had she waited a little longer, her problems would have been resolved spontaneously. Despite all this, Dr. Shead was found guilty—not once, but twice. The answer to this question likely lies in outcome bias, one of the most harmful cognitive biases, as it directly affects how we evaluate the consequences of any action.

Definition

Outcome bias is the flawed cognitive process by which we assess the quality of a decision based on the outcome, without considering the process and analysis that led to it. Thus, favorable or positive outcomes lead us to believe that the right decisions were made, while unfavorable outcomes make us think that a mistake was made in the decision. As with most cognitive biases, a difficult question: how good was my decision? is replaced by a much easier one: what was the result of my decision?

The problem is that evaluating the quality of a decision solely by its consequences does not allow for an adequate assessment of the process that led to it. The outcome of any decision depends on a series of known factors, which are to some extent predictable and even controllable, and on which the decision is based. But the result also depends on other unknown, unforeseen, and random factors over which we have no control, and which are just as decisive and important for the outcome as the known ones. Thus, assuming that every good outcome is the direct result of a good decision is an undeniable cognitive error, since these unknown factors can turn the best decision into the worst outcome, and vice versa.

In Dr. Shead's case, the outcome—a severely diminished and incapacitated patient—was too striking, relevant, and significant to be easily excluded from the analysis of culpability. Thus, when the case went to trial, despite all the arguments presented by the surgeon's defense (extremely rare and already treated complication, successful surgery with ulcer resolution, hasty decision to undergo another procedure which caused the disability, etc.), it was almost impossible to understand and accept that such a disastrous consequence was simply the result of bad luck. There had to be an error on Dr. Shead's part. The consequences are now well known.

History

Outcome bias was described in 1988 by Jonathan Baron and John Hershey at the University of Pennsylvania. In their five experiments, the researchers exposed participants to a series of identical situations (medical, financial and games of chance) in which only the outcome varied, asking them to evaluate the quality of the decision. Additionally, in some groups, they asked which factors had determined their opinion and whether they believed the outcome had influenced it. As illogical as it may seem, depending on the outcome, participants evaluated the quality of the decision in diametrically opposite ways. Good outcomes were considered the result of good decisions, and bad outcomes the result of bad decisions, even though the situations were the same. Even in those entirely determined by chance, such as those related to games of chance, participants continued to believe that their decisions were primarily responsible for the outcomes obtained. To make matters even more complex, when asked whether the outcome had influenced their opinion, virtually no participant considered it relevant (Baron & Hershey, 1988).

Multiple studies have confirmed the initial observations of Baron and Hershey. Among these, the work of Caplan, Posner, and Cheney is of particular relevance to surgeons, as they demonstrated that physicians are especially prone to outcome bias when evaluating the actions of their colleagues and showed that both the severity of judgment and the desire to judge are greater when the outcome is unfavorable (Caplan et al., 1991).

Impact

Life is a constant process of decision-making and outcome evaluation. Therefore, it is expected that the effects of outcome bias extend to all facets of human existence. Among the most important are:

At the Personal Level:

1. **Leads to incorrect and unfair conclusions:** When processes and decisions are evaluated solely by their outcomes, all those unknown and uncontrollable factors that also determine the result of a situation are overlooked. Thus, one may conclude that a certain behavior or approach is correct when it is not or end up blaming a person for a particular error when they are not at fault.
2. **Encourages the blind repetition of past successes:** By considering that every good outcome is the result of a good decision, past actions are automatically repeated in the hope of achieving the same successes, even though these may have been entirely due to luck.
3. **Generates overconfidence and resistance to change:** Achieving good results, attributed to supposedly good decisions, leads to an overestimation of one's abilities and the maintenance of ideas and behaviors that should be changed, either because they are not responsible for the successes or because there are even better alternatives.
4. **Loss of critical analysis of outcomes:** When one becomes accustomed to measuring everything by the outcome, the ability to methodically evaluate processes and decisions is lost and replaced by a simpler, but flawed, approach in which, if the outcome is good, there is no discussion, and if it is bad, someone—usually the decision-maker—is blamed.

At the Collective Level:

1. **Risk aversion, stifling of innovation, and inhibition of growth:** When everything is measured by outcomes and apparent failures are singled out and ridiculed, individuals systematically avoid being associated with them and adopt stable, seemingly safe behaviors that maintain the *status quo* but do not allow for the exploration of new scenarios and possibilities.
2. **Creation of work and social environments where only the outcome matters:** Measuring everything by the outcome generates systematic behaviors aimed at

doing whatever is necessary to achieve good results, to be considered successful and to serve as an example of what should be done, regardless of the collateral losses and damage that such a stance may entail. Controversial and deeply ingrained phrases in society such as "*the end justifies the means*" have their origin in this way of thinking.

Examples in Medical and Surgical Practice

Medicine is a profession where decision-making is constant and, although many decisions are already standardized, critical evaluation of outcomes is an invaluable skill for every medical professional. Unfortunately, outcome bias pervades all areas of medical practice. Among the most significant are:

1. **Incorrect assessment of treatment efficacy,** by allowing the outcome to be the measure through which therapeutic decisions are analyzed. Thus, successful treatments end up being overrated, and effective treatments that, for distinct reasons, did not yield the expected result, end up being discarded. For example, a surgeon who decides to operate on a critically ill patient with a very high probability of mortality: if the patient survives, the surgery was a success and the surgeon a hero, but if the patient dies, the decision was wrong and the surgeon is deemed negligent.
2. **Inappropriate selection of treatments** based on the experience of previous patients, without considering their particular conditions that may have contributed to the treatment's success or failure. For example, a surgeon who always places a voice prosthesis during a total laryngectomy because "*it has always worked for me*," without considering whether the patient meets the cognitive and social criteria for its placement.
3. **Perpetuation of unsuitable behaviors** and even clearly incorrect practices in individual routines and surgical service policies, because "*this is how I've always done it and it has worked for me*." For example, the unnecessary use of prophylactic antibiotics in clean surgical wounds, because "*my patients have never developed infections this way*."
4. **Publication bias in scientific studies:** The desire to highlight successful results extends even to medical literature. Studies with positive results, that is, those where the researchers manage to confirm and/or prove their study hypotheses are published with relative ease, while negative studies, those in which researchers see their hypotheses rejected, achieve relevance and publication much less frequently, regardless of their methodological rigor or even if the negative conclusion is important.
5. **Opinions, evaluations, and assessments by colleagues:** Physicians tend to judge negatively those colleagues who had unfortunate outcomes, without considering the specific circumstances or the process that led to the conduct resulting in unfavorable outcome.

6. **Analysis of medical negligence cases:** in which the diagnostic and therapeutic process is evaluated based on the outcome, and where the degree of culpability depends on the success or failure of the procedure rather than on a reasoned and methodical decision-making process. For example, the previously narrated case.

How to Avoid Falling into This Bias

1. **Learn to evaluate decisions based on the situation and the moment in which they were made:** Instead of focusing on the outcome, ask whether, given the information available at that time, this was the best viable option. Analyze the available data, the known factors, and the reasoning process conducted at that moment.
2. **Document decision-making processes:** Whenever faced with an important and consequential decision, it is advisable to create a record that includes the information used, the alternatives considered, the pros and cons evaluated, and the reasons that led to the selection of a particular option.
3. **Implement structured methodologies:** There are various systems (decision trees, choice matrices, etc.) that provide structure and rigor to the decision-making process, offering a systematic approach to evaluating different options and making better decisions. Learning to use them will make decisions more objective and will later facilitate their evaluation.
4. **Design evaluation plans before conducting the intervention and adhere to them:** Once the decision has been made and well before seeing the results, clearly define the criteria by which it will be evaluated and analyzed. This will help maintain focus on what was important at the time of the decision, preventing the outcome from distorting perception.
5. **Consider alternative scenarios:** Regardless of the outcome, learn to reflect on what would happen if the result had been different, or if another decision had been made, or even if the particular circumstances had been different. This provides context and helps to understand that a good outcome may not have been the result of the best decision.
6. **Take other perspectives:** Ask others to evaluate the decision-making process, especially those who were not involved. During their evaluation, do not disclose the outcome, which will allow for a more objective assessment.

References

Baron, J., & Hershey, J. C. (1988). Outcome bias in decision evaluation. *Journal of Personality and Social Psychology, 54*(4), 569–579. https://doi.org/10.1037//0022-3514.54.4.569
Caplan, R. A., Posner, K. L., & Cheney, F. W. (1991). Effect of outcome on physician judgments of appropriateness of care. *JAMA, 265*(15), 1957–1960. https://www.ncbi.nlm.nih.gov/pubmed/2008024

Hugh, T. B., & Dekker, S. W. (2009). Hindsight bias and outcome bias in the social construction of medical negligence: A review. *Journal of Law and Medicine, 16*(5), 846–857.

Chapter 20
Misinformation Effect: Peptic Ulcer Disease and Gastric Cooling

The Problem

In 1959, Owen Hardin Wangensteen, a surgeon at the University of Minnesota and a prominent academic known for his role in the development of cardiac surgery, presented his experiments on the rate of food digestion in a native stomach subjected to hypothermia. Studies conducted in animal models showed that the digestive process slowed for hours when stomachs were kept at low temperatures. Subsequently, the experiments were replicated in humans with comparable results: the weight of a meat sample decreased by 55% in a stomach at normal temperatures, while it decreased by only 18% when the stomach was kept at temperatures close to 11 degrees Celsius. Gastric hypothermia also reduced gastric secretion by 80–90% (Wangensteen et al., 1962a).

With this in mind, Wangensteen designed a homemade gastric cooling machine in collaboration with the Swenko company, which included a multi-lumen nasogastric tube with a balloon, through which ethyl alcohol was continuously instilled, maintaining a constant temperature of 0 to 2 °C for about 48h. Once completed, he began using it as a strategy to treat massive bleeding from peptic ulcers or esophageal varices. In some patients, the procedure also included prophylactic tracheostomy to prevent bronchial aspiration of gastric contents. Gastric cooling was maintained until the return from the nasogastric tube was clear and there was no evidence of active bleeding. By 1962, he had already documented successful treatment in 120 patients, reporting achlorhydria in most of them after treatment; thus, by October of that year, Wangensteen decided to expand his treatment with even lower temperatures, between −10 and −20 °C (gastric freezing), to patients with non-bleeding ulcers, proposing the concept of "*physiological gastrectomy*" (Wangensteen et al., 1962b). Over time, the indications for the therapy were broadened to other conditions such as intractable duodenal ulcer, post-gastrectomy ulcer, and it was even used as a preventive method for stress ulcers, with apparently promising results in 387 patients who underwent the therapy (Bernstein et al., 1963; McFee et al., 1963).

A. Sanabria and C. Betancourt, *Cognitive Biases in Surgical Practice*,
https://doi.org/10.1007/978-3-032-20377-9_20

With these results, by 1963 the first cases were performed in France, Argentina, Brazil and the United Kingdom, and the technique quickly spread to other European countries thanks to the accessibility provided by its inventors and the ease of its implementation. It was even proposed as an outpatient procedure. The magazines *Time* and *Readers Digest* published brief notes on the treatment, and there were favorable media reports on radio and television (4 minute read, 1963).

Nevertheless, in 1963 the first warnings about adverse events from gastric freezing emerged, and in 1964 the first external evaluations appeared, showing a lower success rate than previously reported. Herbert Livingston Duthie (Duthie, 1964), a surgeon at the General Infirmary at Leeds, UK, published a strong critique of Wangensteen's results, suggesting that the effects of gastric freezing were transient and disappeared after six months. Paradoxically, Wangensteen's own son, Stephen Lightner Wangensteen, became one of the strongest critics of gastric freezing as a treatment for duodenal ulcers, leaving open the option of using gastric cooling only for massive bleeding (Wangensteen et al., 1966). Despite this, the number of procedures performed in the United States continued to rise, as did the production and purchase of freezing devices (Gilbertson, 1964).

Finally, Julian Ruffin from Duke University, in 1969 published a multicenter clinical trial demonstrated that gastric freezing offered no advantage in the treatment of duodenal ulcer (Ruffin et al., 1969). Nevertheless, Wangensteen and his group continued to advocate for the benefits of the treatment well into the 1970s (Ritchie et al., 1966). In his memoir, *The Rise of Surgery: From Empiric Craft to Scientific Discipline*, he referenced his technique, despite the substantial and compelling evidence demonstrating its lack of efficacy. Likewise, Wilye Gibbons, an Australian surgeon who worked with Wangensteen, published a book on the method in 2017 *(Gastric Hypothermia for Major Haematemesis: The Practicable Use of Gastric Cooling to Treat Gastrointestinal Bleeding Incorporating Investigation, New Methodology and Clinical Aspects)* (Gibbons, 2017). Thus, the technique of gastric freezing was not completely abandoned until the advent and development of H2 inhibitors and the discovery of the role of *H. pylori* in the pathogenesis of the disease. However, despite the controversy surrounding the technique and its inadequate results, it is estimated that 2,500 cooling machines were sold and between 15,000 and 25,000 patients were treated in the United States alone (Council & Medicine, 1979).

The question that arises more than 50 years later is how the use of gastric freezing could have become so widespread. While it was effective for the management of massive gastric hemorrhage, its use beyond this indication was controversial and very limited, not to mention the complications and adverse effects. Even more concerning is how Wangensteen could continue to defend and promote its use when it was clear that the results did not support it. The answer likely lies in the misinformation effect, one of the cognitive biases that most dangerously affect memory.

Definition

Misinformation can be defined as the dissemination of unverified information that occurs unintentionally, distinguishing it from disinformation, which is planned and intentional.

The misinformation effect is the tendency to alter a memory with new information acquired after the event, leading to the modification of memories or even the creation of new ones. This phenomenon is part of a broader concept known as *retroactive interference*, which occurs when recently acquired information interferes with the ability to retain and recall previously encoded information.

Two explanations have been proposed to account for the misinformation effect:

1. The inadvertent combination of new information with memories, or their replacement, due to a misattribution of the information to an internal source (one's own memories) when in fact the source is external (exogenous information).
2. Each time a memory is retrieved, it may be modified by new information, as the added information is more recent and easier to recall. This new information can alter original memories or even fill in gaps (confabulation).

It is also known that children and the elderly, individuals with reduced working memory, and those with certain personality traits (introversion, empathy, cooperativeness, and sensitivity to negative peer evaluation) are more susceptible to the effect. Additionally, the source of the misinformation (credibility, authority), the temporal distance from the event (the more distant, the more powerful), the subject's mental model (misinformation that fits the model is more easily accepted), and repetition (multiple episodes of misinformation, varied sources) can promote the establishment and persistence of misinformation.

There are several factors that facilitate the spread of misinformation:

1. The anxiety of the recipient. Higher anxiety increases the likelihood of spreading rumors.
2. Excessive trust in the source of erroneous information, whether due to authority or social proximity.
3. The personal impact of the information on the recipient (personal memories, involvement in related events), where greater self-identification increases the likelihood of dissemination.
4. The aesthetics of the information, with products featuring more elaborate graphics or audio elements being more likely to be disseminated.
5. Individual traits in relation to the type of information received. People with greater sensitivity to visual elements may be more likely to alter their memory in response to a photograph, compared to those more sensitive to verbal elements.
6. The interval between the original memory and the acquisition of new information. The more distant the memory, the more likely it is that erroneous added information will be accepted.
7. The use of narratives. If new information is presented within more elaborate and complex narratives, it is more likely to be accepted.

As described, Wangensteen conducted experiments and firmly believed in the advantages of his technique, published his data, and engaged in academic discussion and debate. Although his results were incorrect, he never intended to provide false information, which rules out disinformation. He demonstrated the utility of his gastric cooling technique in a specific population of critically ill patients at high surgical risk and with massive gastric bleeding, with the aim of stopping the critical episode and providing a window of time to consider other treatments. However, the initial results showed utility in other conditions (new information). Thus, he modified his original technique by further lowering the temperature (freezing) to apply it to another patient population, those with duodenal ulcers, with a different goal: to treat peptic ulcer disease. In this transition, he altered his initial approach (previous information) and conveyed his erroneous information to a significant number of surgeons in North America, South America, and Europe, involving the industry to design gastric freezing devices, which were commercialized and used by multiple hospitals and in a considerable number of patients. Analysis of Wangensteen's studies shows the progressive modification of his initial intentions, focused on patients with massive hematemesis, as he accumulated data, shaping his idea of using the same technique to treat different diseases. Furthermore, there is evidence of his active defense of his proposal and resistance to acknowledging contradictory data. In the end, he seemed to have forgotten that the original objective of the procedure was massive gastric hemorrhage, acting as if the evidence originally obtained applied to the new indications, when this was clearly not the case.

History

Memory has been a subject of interest since the origins of human thought. Herodotus and Thucydides, the great Greek historians, relied on memory to preserve the achievements of humanity. For a long time, memory was assumed to be unchangeable and unalterable, like a paper on which one writes, and which does not allow modifications.

In 1932, Sir Frederic Bartlett (Bartlett, 1995), psychologist and director of the psychology laboratory at the University of Cambridge, published his most famous work, *Remembering*, in which he changed the concept of memory as a fixed and static faculty and paved the way for the acceptance of the constructive nature of memory. Today, it is accepted that memory is a process of reconstructing events, not a recorder, and is vulnerable to both internal and external influences (Chan et al., 2017).

In 1974, Elizabeth Loftus (Zagorski, 2005), psychologist at the Department of Psychology at the University of Washington, published a study demonstrating that the way questions are designed to elicit a memory can modify it. Using 45 subjects, she showed that associating the description of a car accident with the word "*smash*" led subjects to estimate a higher speed than when more neutral words like "*hit*" were used (Loftus & Palmer, 1974). In 1978, a second study in which a stop sign was replaced with a yield sign in an image of a car accident demonstrated that introducing new information about a memory modifies it. This gave rise to what is now known as the "*misinformation effect.*" It is now accepted that memory has weaknesses that make it susceptible to errors such as *suggestibility*, which is the influence that information and interactions with others exert on our own memories, and *misattribution*, which involves adopting information from exogenous sources as our own memories (Byrne, 2017).

The consequences of identifying the misinformation effect were immediately seen in the administration of justice. Since many trials depended on eyewitnesses, research showed that witnesses were prone to both extrinsic and intrinsic modifications of their memories of the events about which they testified. This research was later expanded, evaluating the possibility of implanting false memories in people; it was shown that, in some cases of hypnosis, false memories could be planted by therapists and later used in court. In recent decades, Loftus and her team demonstrated that, because of the misinformation effect, voter preferences can be altered (Loftus, 2005).

Impact

The misinformation effect has been identified in multiple aspects of modern life. It occurs preferentially in relation to political events, health, and disasters. The influence of social media in the 2016 US elections or the attribution of the spread of the COVID-19 virus to certain ethnic groups are well-known examples of the effects of misinformation.

At the Personal Level:

False Associations Driving Public Health Decline. In health, the case of the false association between the measles vaccine and autism, which gave rise to the anti-vaccine movement, has reduced the use of other vaccines with proven effectiveness.

At the Collective Level:

Misinformation's Impact on Decisions, Outcomes, and Trust. Today, social media are the main, though not the only, disseminators of misinformation. Its effects can be seen in terms of poor choices (decision-makers opting for less effective alternatives), loss of life and quality of life (people who do not access correct information and avoid effective treatments, or those who, due to incorrect information, undergo ineffective treatments), economic losses (investment in treatments with dubious or negative outcomes), and loss of trust (acceptance of opinions and recommendations from pseudo-associations or *influencers* without support in valid scientific evidence, leading to resistance to recommendations from governmental or scientific institutions).

Examples in Practice

The effect of misinformation has existed throughout history of medicine. Although it has recently become a problem of significant proportions, due to the rise of social media and the ease of sharing information among peers. Some examples that demonstrate its presence in surgical culture include:

1. **Recommendations from physician "*influencers*" without specialized training in a particular field**: These individuals disseminate concepts that may be useful in certain areas of surgery, but not in others. This information can alter the pre-existing concepts of other surgeons. For example, in a study on sinusitis, up to 16% of healthcare professionals shared videos containing erroneous information (Dimitroyannis et al., 2024).
2. **The rise of "predatory" journals**: These journals publish information that has not undergone peer review. It has been identified that a substantial number of surgical journals fit the definition of predatory journals, where the methodological quality of studies is low or deficient and whose conclusions are of questionable applicability in daily practice (Moher et al., 2017). This new and usually free information can affect physicians' understanding and lead them to make mistakes.
3. **Memory Distortion Through Shared Narratives**. In error analysis meetings, adverse event reviews, or complication discussions, the versions that are shared and discussed beforehand among those involved in the case can alter individual recollections of the event. This is similar to what has been demonstrated in legal cases with eyewitnesses, where testimonies are modified as they are shared and discussed.
4. **The use of extrinsic sources such as "opinion *leaders*"**: Individuals who have financial or non-financial conflicts of interest, potentially influencing surgeons' decision-making. There is evidence suggesting that opinion leaders who receive sponsorship and payments from industry tend to favor certain therapeutic alternatives. If this information is disseminated, it can alter the decision-making processes of other surgeons.

How to Avoid Falling into Bias

1. **Early communication and anticipation**: When facing a phenomenon that can be anticipated as susceptible to misinformation, the early production and dissemination of accurate information and prominent warnings about misinformation are useful, provided these are highly visible and issued before exposure (prebunking). Those issued afterward are often ineffective or even counterproductive. For example, in the context of a potential piece of information presented at a surgical congress promoting a new device that has not yet been evaluated in randomized clinical trials, it is possible to provide advance information to warn surgeons about the seriousness or strength of claims regarding the device (Ecker et al., 2022).

2. **Providing information to correct misinformation (Debunking):** This is defined as offering a message that identifies another message as partially or totally misinformative. It should be detailed, should not repeat the arguments of the misinformation, and must specify which data is incorrect by comparing them with the correct information (Chan et al., 2017). A variant of this approach is the so-called *fact-checking report*, which evaluates claims point by point and gives them a seal of approval or disapproval. Another alternative is the design of *accuracy prompts*, which are messages attached to potentially erroneous information, asking the reader whether they believe the information is true or false and whether it is worth sharing. For example, in response to sensationalist or promotional press reports, academic institutions, scientific associations, and surgeons themselves can issue clarifying statements about what is true and what is not.
3. **Use reliable sources**: Sources that contradict misinformation should be highly reliable, with an authoritative reputation that is difficult to discredit and ideally supported by other voices with similar credibility.
4. **Keep records**: In situations where a high degree of influence from new information is expected, written or audiovisual records allow comparison of this added information with the original. For example, video recordings of endoscopic surgeries are an effective method for evaluating complications and are resistant to the effects of misinformation.

References

4 minute read. (1963, November 8). Medicine: To freeze or not to freeze? *Time*. https://time.com/archive/6832021/medicine-to-freeze-or-not-to-freeze/

Bartlett, F. C. (1995). *Remembering: A study in experimental and social psychology*. Cambridge University Press. https://books.google.com.co/books?id=WG5ZcHGTrm4C

Bernstein, E. F., Mc, F. A., Goodale, R. L., Jr., Madsen, A. J., & Wangensteen, O. H. (1963). Treatment of postgastrectomy stomal ulcer by gastric freezing. *Archives of Surgery, 87*, 13–22. https://doi.org/10.1001/archsurg.1963.01310130015003

Byrne, J. H. (2017). *Learning and memory: A comprehensive reference*. Elsevier Science. https://books.google.com.co/books?id=QhNvDgAAQBAJ

Chan, M. S., Jones, C. R., Hall Jamieson, K., & Albarracin, D. (2017). Debunking: A meta-analysis of the psychological efficacy of messages countering misinformation. *Psychological Science, 28*(11), 1531–1546. https://doi.org/10.1177/0956797617714579

Council, N. R., & Medicine, I. o. (1979). *Medical technology and the health care system: A study of the diffusion of equipment-embodied technology*. The National Academies Press. https://doi.org/10.17226/18439

Dimitroyannis, R., Fenton, D., Cho, S., Nordgren, R., Pinto, J. M., & Roxbury, C. R. (2024). A social media quality review of popular sinusitis videos on TikTok. *Otolaryngology—Head and Neck Surgery, 170*(5), 1456–1466. https://doi.org/10.1002/ohn.688

Duthie, H. L. (1964). Gastric freezing for duodenal ulcer. *Postgraduate Medical Journal, 40*(461), 120–124. https://doi.org/10.1136/pgmj.40.461.120

Ecker, U. K. H., Lewandowsky, S., Cook, J., Schmid, P., Fazio, L. K., Brashier, N., Kendeou, P., Vraga, E. K., & Amazeen, M. A. (2022). The psychological drivers of misinformation belief and its resistance to correction. *Nature Reviews Psychology, 1*(1), 13–29. https://doi.org/10.1038/s44159-021-00006-y

Gibbons, W. (2017). *Gastric hypothermia* (1st Ed.). Gibbons Publishing.

Gilbertson, R. B. (1964). Gastric freezing. *JAMA, 187*, 1032–1033. https://doi.org/10.1001/jama.1964.03060260060023

Loftus, E. F. (2005). Planting misinformation in the human mind: A 30-year investigation of the malleability of memory. *Learning & Memory, 12*(4), 361–366. https://doi.org/10.1101/lm.94705

Loftus, E. F., & Palmer, J. C. (1974). *Reconstruction of automobile destruction: An example of the interaction between language and memory.* https://doi.org/10.1016/S0022-5371(74)80011-3. Elsevier Science.

McFee, A. S., Stone, N. H., Goodale, R. L., Jr., Bernstein, E. F., & Wangensteen, O. H. (1963). Prevention of stress-induced ulcer in the rat by gastric freezing. A study showing protection afforded rats whose stomachs had been frozen. *JAMA, 186*, 917–919. https://doi.org/10.1001/jama.1963.63710100001013

Moher, D., Shamseer, L., Cobey, K. D., Lalu, M. M., Galipeau, J., Avey, M. T., Ahmadzai, N., Alabousi, M., Barbeau, P., Beck, A., Daniel, R., Frank, R., Ghannad, M., Hamel, C., Hersi, M., Hutton, B., Isupov, I., McGrath, T. A., McInnes, M. D. F., & Ziai, H. et al. (2017). Stop this waste of people, animals and money. *Nature, 549*(7670), 23–25. https://doi.org/10.1038/549023a

Ritchie, W. P., Jr., Edlich, R. F., Breen, J. J., Molina, J. E., & Wangensteen, O. H. (1966). Experimental and clinical experience with gastric freezing. *JAMA, 198*(3), 237–242.

Ruffin, J. M., Grizzle, J. E., Hightower, N. C., McHardy, G., Shull, H., & Kirsner, J. B. (1969). A cooperative double-blind evaluation of gastric "freezing" in the treatment of duodenal ulcer. *New England Journal of Medicine, 281*(1), 16–19. https://doi.org/10.1056/NEJM196907032810104

Wangensteen, O. H., Peter, E. T., Bernstein, E. F., Walder, A. I., Sosin, H., & Madsen, A. J. (1962a). Can physiological gastrectomy be achieved by gastric freezing? *Annals of Surgery, 156*(4), 579–591. https://doi.org/10.1097/00000658-196210000-00006

Wangensteen, O. H., Peter, E. T., Nicoloff, D. M., Walder, A. I., Sosin, H., & Bernstein, E. F. (1962b). Achieving "physiological gastrectomy" by gastric freezing. A preliminary report of an experimental and clinical study. *JAMA, 180*, 439–444. https://doi.org/10.1001/jama.1962.03050190001001

Wangensteen, S. L., Smith, R. B., 3rd., & Barker, H. G. (1966). Gastric cooling and gastric "freezing." *Surgical Clinics of North America, 46*(2), 463–475. https://doi.org/10.1016/s0039-6109(16)37847-1

Zagorski, N. (2005). Profile of Elizabeth F. Loftus. *Proc Natl Acad Sci U S A, 102* (39), 13721–13723. https://doi.org/10.1073/pnas.0506223102

Chapter 21
The Framing Effect: Bernard Fisher and the New Paradigm of Mastectomy

The Problem

In the late nineteenth and early twentieth centuries, breast cancer was an indolent disease with few treatment options. Most patients requested medical attention only at advanced stages, due to a combination of factors such as the social stigma associated with exposing intimate body parts (even to physicians), lack of understanding of disease progression, the belief that cancer was a divine punishment to be accepted with resignation, and a justified fear of surgery, which was performed without the benefits of general anesthesia, carried high mortality due to infections in the pre-antiseptic era, and resulted in bodily defects that could not be adequately reconstructed (Ekmektzoglou et al., 2009). These were patients with tumors that could only be palliated, whose deaths were painful and humiliating, resulting from a combination of locoregional and systemic disease.

In this context, William Halsted (Fig. 21.1), a surgeon at Johns Hopkins University considered the father of modern American surgery, proposed his strategy of radical mastectomy (removal of the mammary gland, underlying muscles, and axillary lymph nodes) for the treatment of breast cancer at the end of the nineteenth century (Imber, 2010). At the time, Halsted's approach was based on established clinical observation and anatomical knowledge, which explained cancer progression as a sequential process that began locally and spread in an orderly fashion to regional lymph nodes and then to other parts of the body. In this framework, a large and extensive surgery could control advanced disease, thereby preventing systemic spread and death. Although increased survival was never proven, radical mastectomy demonstrated its advantages in terms of reducing local disease recurrence after surgery. However, this success came at the cost of severe sequelae such as chronic swelling of the affected arm, physical disability due to removal of the pectoral muscles, and resulting physical deformities. As a result, radical mastectomy, including extended variants that even removed parts of the chest wall, became the standard of care for breast cancer (Cotlar et al., 2003).

A. Sanabria and C. Betancourt, *Cognitive Biases in Surgical Practice*,
https://doi.org/10.1007/978-3-032-20377-9_21

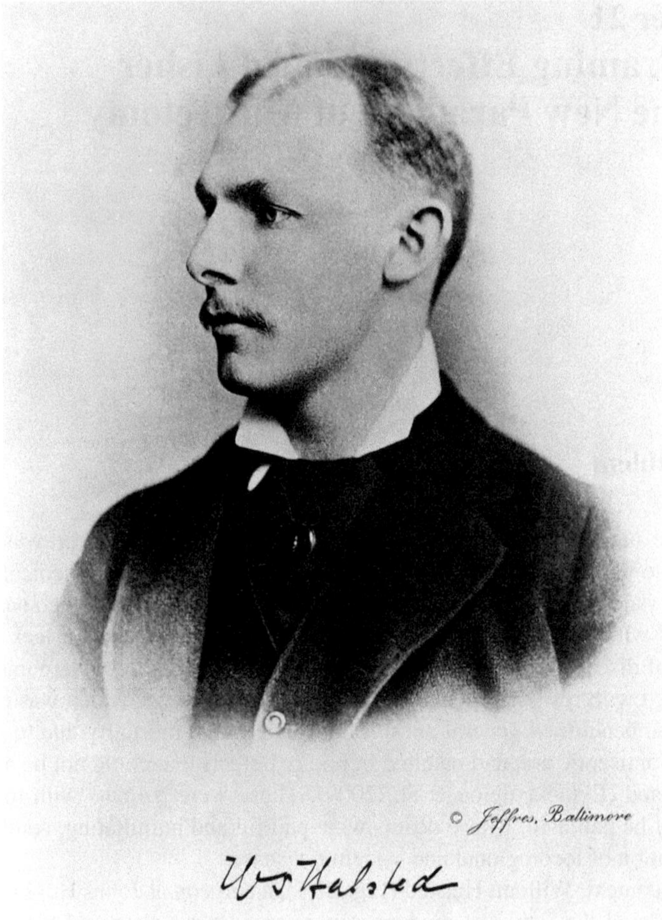

Fig. 21.1 William Halsted, surgeon who designed the classic radical mastectomy (Public domain). Portrait of William Stewart Halsted. Library reference: Slide number 6263. Photo number: M0012697. Full Bibliographic Record: http://catalogue.wellcomelibrary.org/record=b1323063

In the mid-twentieth century, Bernard Fisher (Fisher & Anderson, 2010), another surgeon from the University of Pittsburgh (Fig. 21.2), challenged Halsted's thesis, which had remained unquestionable for several decades as the cornerstone of breast cancer treatment, when he designed the landmark clinical trials of the National Surgical Adjuvant Breast and Bowel Project (NSABP). Fisher conducted a series of clinical experiments, recruiting patients from multiple cancer centers worldwide, to demonstrate that the extent of surgery did not improve cure rates and that, even with less mutilating procedures, disease control comparable to that of the time could be achieved, with a lower proportion of physical, functional, and aesthetic adverse effects. The new paradigm proposed that breast cancer was a systemic disease that did not follow the rigid dissemination laws proposed by Halsted and that, with a combination of treatments such as radiotherapy and chemotherapy alongside much less extensive surgery (quadrantectomy), better outcomes could be obtained (Fisher, 1992). This generated criticism, lawsuits, and opposition from the surgical community and society at large (Carpenter & Twedt, 2019). Nevertheless, despite initial rejection, Fisher and the group at the United States National Cancer Institute succeeded in changing the treatment paradigm. In the end, after several years of follow-up, the data proved that Fisher was right.

In addition to the evidence supporting his proposals, Fisher's group succeeded in changing the perception of treatment thanks to a change in the way results were presented. While Halsted's proponents focused on locoregional control (Klem, 2013), Fisher's supporters emphasized overall survival (Schuller, 2006). The former highlighted the risk of leaving residual tumor when using less aggressive surgery, which could result in more metastases, whereas the latter focused on the functional and aesthetic advantages of the new procedure, which preserved the breast and avoided the consequences of limb edema and impaired mobility. While some invoked Halsted's

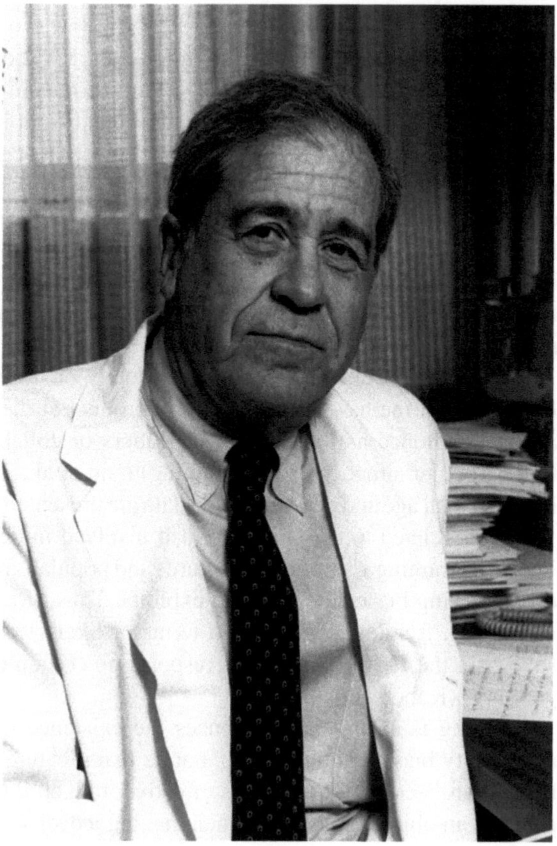

Fig. 21.2 Bernard Fisher. Surgeon and pioneer of modern breast surgery (public domain)

authority as the father of American surgery, others stressed trust in the scientific method far beyond individual recognition. The former defended their position from the physician's perspective, while the latter chose to view the problem from the standpoint of women affected by the disease. Although the work was not easy and it took more than two decades for the approach to be widely accepted and practiced, Fisher's breast-conserving surgery prevailed.

Currently, radical mastectomies based on Halsted's principles are obsolete. Breast-conserving surgery is the gold standard in the surgical management of breast cancer. The results were simply too overwhelming to maintain the initial approach. However, changing the paradigm required a shift in how information was communicated. The question that arises today is why this was necessary. Such compelling evidence should have been sufficient to bring about change. Yet, this was not the case. How, then, can this be explained? The answer likely lies in the framing effect, one of the most important cognitive biases when evaluating the world around us.

Definition

It is well known that people interpret the world according to a frame of reference based on their subjective opinions, a kind of mental structure that allows them to determine what is relevant and meaningful and what is not (Beratšová et al., 2016).

The framing effect is a mental phenomenon that occurs when decisions and evaluations vary depending on how the characteristics of certain information are presented, even when the information is identical in terms of benefits and risks. The bias, therefore, does not depend on the information itself, but on the way that information is brought to attention. Thus, situations or choices presented as positive (gains) will be accepted by people, while those presented as negative (losses) will be rejected, regardless of whether they are two sides of the same coin.

The framing effect can occur individually or in groups, and its impact may be limited, as in the case of purchasing a product at the supermarket, or widespread, as when it concerns the election of leaders or collaborative activities in response to a particular situation (social framing) (Liu et al., 2020). Moreover, it appears to increase with age and decrease when data are presented in a non-native language, both situations related to the cognitive load involved in decision-making. Similarly, the impact of framing varies across cultures and populations, explained by the prevalence of underlying biases that framing exploits. Thus, if loss aversion is more prevalent in a group, framing a proposal in terms of likely losses will have a greater effect. Likewise, the bias is stronger in response to certain external stimuli (such as time pressure) (Roberts et al., 2022).

Framing is a bias that influences the existence of other biases (loss aversion, availability bias, negativity bias), but its main feature is that it organizes how these biases can become more or less effective, reducing the cognitive load required to perform an objective analysis when making a decision.

Several ways of classifying framing have been proposed: (Piñon & Gambara, 2005).

A. **Choice**, when information is presented in a way that favors one of the options: positively (favorable outcomes), promoting the safer option, or negatively (unfavorable outcomes), promoting the less risky option.
B. **Attribution**: when the information presented highlights a particular characteristic of an object or person to favor an option positively (advantages) with the intention of it being chosen, or negatively (disadvantages) so that it is rejected.
C. **Action**: when the information emphasizes the consequences of choosing a particular option by visualizing gains (chances of success) or losses (chances of failure), with the aim of prompting a specific behavior.

In turn, framing bias may involve the information itself or contextual aspects such as auditory cues (e.g., when a message is heard and its syntax, tone, volume, etc., are modified), visual cues (e.g., changes in color, font, environment, etc.), or the messenger (e.g., changing the source by using profession, prominence, or authority). Additionally, factors such as the order in which options are presented and the number of options (the greater the number of options, the better the decisions) affect the choice.

In the story described, it was the change in framing that helped the new alternative of breast-conserving mastectomy gain the prominence it has today. Halsted's approach emphasized the negative aspects of conservative treatment (local recurrence, risk of residual tumor), while Fisher's approach highlighted its positive aspects (breast preservation, improved function and aesthetics). When faced with a surgical procedure that entails risks (mastectomy) and in an environment of uncertainty (local vs. systemic control, sequelae, etc.), the way results were presented significantly influenced how physicians and patients approached the decision and the final position they assumed regarding it.

History

In logic, it is accepted that two propositions with the same conditions and the same truth value can be interchangeable, a principle known as extensionality. This implies that regardless of how the propositions are presented, the derived conclusion should be the same. This is one of the arguments supporting the idea of the *homo economicus*, a rational individual who makes decisions looking to optimize their utility.

In 1979, Amos Tversky and Daniel Kahneman proposed their prospect theory of decision-making and introduced the framing effect with an example related to medicine (the Asian disease problem), where they offered treatment alternatives, one focused on survival and the other on mortality (Tversky & Kahneman, 1981). In their study, they demonstrated that decision-makers were more sensitive to losses than to gains, which led people to choose the safer options in each scenario (the safe alternative in gain scenarios and the less safe alternatives in loss scenarios).

In 1991, Valerie Reyna and Charles Brainerd, psychologists at the University of Arizona, (Reyna & Brainerd, 1991) proposed the *Fuzzy-trace theory*, which suggests that the cognitive load associated with decision-making is a relevant factor, as people tend to opt for decisions that are less complex and require fewer cognitive resources.

Other motivational approaches have suggested that individuals make decisions based on the hedonic forces (fears and desires) associated with the choice, favoring those that provide more pleasure or less discomfort (Lopes, 1987).

In 1998, Irvin Levin, Sandra Schneider, and Gary Gaetth proposed the currently accepted taxonomy of framing bias, dividing it into its types: *risky choice, attribute, and goal (*Levin et al., 1998*).*

Impact

Traditionally, the framing effect has been used in the world of marketing and advertising, where a product with the same characteristics is presented in a positive way (emphasizing its advantages) or a negative way (emphasizing its weaknesses), influencing and guiding the person toward the desired or expected choice. The most common examples are the presentation of a product, where one of its features is prominently highlighted without mentioning its disadvantages or only mentioning them marginally (for example, highlighting the modern design of a vehicle but not its fuel consumption); or presenting only information on certain sensitive topics while omitting others (for example, media advertising of a political candidate's proposals that are favorable on economic issues while omitting controversial topics such as those related to health). There are also non-binary alternatives to framing, such as interposing a choice between two options with extreme conditions, which shifts the selection toward one of the options (for example, when a service subscription offers a low, a high, and an extremely high option, pushing the choice toward the middle one).

Similarly, focusing the audience's attention on how arguments are expressed rather than their content can mask reasons that act for or against a particular course of action. Thus, framing can facilitate manipulation if the goal is to obtain personal or social benefit from the decision, but it can also facilitate the achievement of goals if the aim is to promote the adoption of beneficial behaviors. Beyond marketing, the framing effect is observed in all disciplines, such as law, finance, and medicine.

Examples in Medical and Surgical Practice

Framing bias has been widely studied in medicine. In fact, its original description is closely linked to a problem of option selection in a clinical context (the Asian disease problem). Thus, its potential effects are expected to be broad and diverse. Among the most important are:

1. **Biased indication of interventions and/or treatments:** Only mentioning the potential benefits of a particular surgery or drug, without mentioning its possible adverse effects or sequelae. For example, mentioning only the advantages of laparoscopic cholecystectomy in the treatment of Acute Cholecystitis, while omitting the potential risks of surgery or other treatment alternatives.
2. **Promoting preventive activities** by presenting adverse outcomes, such as the use of sunscreen described as preventing the development of skin cancer (Morris et al., 2014).
3. **Encouraging healthy behaviors** by presenting only the benefits, such as exercise in obese individuals to achieve improvements in blood glucose or cholesterol levels (Correa & Tabak, 2024).
4. **Promoting certain activities or behaviors:** By making susceptibility to a certain condition visible as a mechanism to introduce framed information. For example, conducting a breast cancer awareness campaign to then introduce the use of screening mammography with positive outcomes such as breast preservation.
5. **Favoring the choice of specific surgical alternatives**: By presenting options in absolute terms, making a riskier option more attractive compared to when options are presented in relative terms. For example, stating that surgical treatment offers a twofold greater chance of survival is more accepted than when it is said that the chance of survival increases from 10 to 20%.

It is accepted that framing bias consistently influences medical decision-making, but in some cases, it may operate in the opposite direction: in positively framed scenarios, the risky option is preferred, while in negatively framed scenarios, the safe option is chosen (Gong et al., 2013).

How to Avoid It

1. **Acquire knowledge about the topic under discussion:** Immersion and in-depth understanding of a particular subject make individuals less susceptible to bias. When faced with information from mass media or scientific journals, a person who has studied the topic will be less likely to be influenced by framing.
2. **Use tools that facilitate rational decision-making:** When deciding, use available instruments (decision trees, flowcharts, checklists) to incorporate relevant information about the problem and enable a balanced evaluation of the options, thereby reducing the influence of bias.
3. **Rebalance:** When data are presented in favor of or against a decision, use the complement of the data and reanalyze the decision. For example, if a medication is reported to have a 70% effectiveness rate, reorganize the information by considering that it has a 30% failure rate and reconsider your choice.
4. **Peer review:** When deciding, include stakeholders with divergent perspectives who are considered independent and highly credible. Each will have different frames of reference, allowing the decision to be evaluated from a more neutral

standpoint. For example, when purchasing a supply, include administrative staff as well as operational personnel and end users.

5. **Embed negative information within a positive message:** This method, known as "*two-side framing*," in which a small amount of negative information is included within a positive message, helps protect against bias. For example, when discussing a surgical procedure, focus on the success rate but also introduce data on the most relevant risks and their magnitude to provide transparency and credibility.
6. **Challenge the false dilemma:** When faced with a range of possible decisions, two alternatives are often presented as the only options, usually clearly framed. In these scenarios, consider a third or even more alternatives. For example, when deciding between surgery or medical management for a specific condition (such as asymptomatic inguinal hernia), opting for temporary observation can help reconsider the available choices.

References

Beratšová, A., Krchová, K., Gažová, N., & Jirásek, M. (2016). Framing and bias: A literature review of recent findings. *Central European Journal of Management, 3*(2), 23–32.

Carpenter, M., & Twedt, S. (2019, November 1). Anatomy of a scandal. *The Cancer Letter*, *45*(1). https://cancerletter.com/the-cancer-letter/20191101_2/

Correa, R., & Tabak, B. M. (2024). The influence of behavioral sciences on adherence to physical activity and weight loss in overweight and obese patients: A systematic review of randomized controlled trials. *Int J Environ Res Public Health, 21*(5). https://doi.org/10.3390/ijerph21050630

Cotlar, A. M., Dubose, J. J., & Rose, D. M. (2003). History of surgery for breast cancer: Radical to the sublime. *Current Surgery, 60*(3), 329–337. https://doi.org/10.1016/S0149-7944(02)00777-8

Ekmektzoglou, K. A., Xanthos, T., German, V., & Zografos, G. C. (2009). Breast cancer: From the earliest times through to the end of the 20th century. *European Journal of Obstetrics, Gynecology, and Reproductive Biology, 145*(1), 3–8. https://doi.org/10.1016/j.ejogrb.2009.03.017

Fisher, B. (1992). The evolution of paradigms for the management of breast cancer: A personal perspective1. *Cancer Research, 52*(9), 2371–2383.

Fisher, B., & Anderson, S. J. (2010). The breast cancer alternative hypothesis: Is there evidence to justify replacing it? *Journal of Clinical Oncology, 28*(3), 366–374. https://doi.org/10.1200/JCO.2009.26.8292

Gong, J., Zhang, Y., Yang, Z., Huang, Y., Feng, J., & Zhang, W. (2013). The framing effect in medical decision-making: A review of the literature. *Psychology, Health & Medicine, 18*(6), 645–653. https://doi.org/10.1080/13548506.2013.766352

Imber, G. (2010). *Genius on the edge: The Bizarre double life of Dr. William Stewart Halsted*. Kaplan Publishing. https://books.google.com.co/books?id=kdUhAQAAMAAJ

Klem, J. (2013). Framing the debate: The trends in mastectomy rates. *Am J Managed Care, 19*(sp4), sp134. https://www.ajmc.com/view/framing-the-debate-the-trends-in-mastectomy-rates

Levin, I. P., Schneider, S. L., & Gaeth, G. J. (1998). *All frames are not created equal: A typology and critical analysis of framing effects* https://doi.org/10.1006/obhd.1998.2804. Elsevier Science.

Liu, J., Gu, R., Liao, C., Lu, J., Fang, Y., Xu, P., Luo, Y. J., & Cui, F. (2020). The neural mechanism of the social framing effect: Evidence from fMRI and tDCS studies. *Journal of Neuroscience, 40*(18), 3646–3656. https://doi.org/10.1523/JNEUROSCI.1385-19.2020

Lopes, L. L. (1987). Between hope and fear: The psychology of risk. In L. Berkowitz (Ed.), *Advances in experimental social psychology* (Vol. 20, pp. 255–295). Academic Press. https://doi.org/10.1016/S0065-2601(08)60416-5

Morris, K. L., Cooper, D. P., Goldenberg, J. L., Arndt, J., & Gibbons, F. X. (2014). Improving the efficacy of appearance-based sun exposure interventions with the terror management health model. *Psychology & Health, 29*(11), 1245–1264. https://doi.org/10.1080/08870446.2014.922184

Piñon, A., & Gambara, H. (2005). A meta-analytic review of framing effect: Risky, attribute and goal framing. *Psicothema, 17*(2), 325–331.

Reyna, V. F., & Brainerd, C. J. (1991). Fuzzy-trace theory and framing effects in choice: Gist extraction, truncation, and conversion. *Journal of Behavioral Decision Making, 4*(4), 249–262. https://doi.org/10.1002/bdm.3960040403

Roberts, I. D., Teoh, Y. Y., & Hutcherson, C. A. (2022). Time to pay attention? Information Search explains amplified framing effects under time pressure. *Psychological Science, 33*(1), 90–104. https://doi.org/10.1177/09567976211026983

Schuller, K. (2006). *The framing effect and breast cancer treatment options: Do individual characteristics play a role?* (Publication Number 4265). West Virginia University. Morgantown, West Virginia. https://researchrepository.wvu.edu/etd/4265

Tversky, A., & Kahneman, D. (1981). The framing of decisions and the psychology of choice. *Science, 211*(4481), 453–458. https://doi.org/10.1126/science.7455683

Chapter 22
Survivorship Bias: Battey and Normal Ovariotomy

The Problem

In 1851, the renowned writer Charles Dickens visited St Luke's Hospital for the Insane in London. There, he discovered that of the 18,759 patients the institution had received during its existence, 11,162 had been women. After his visit, he wrote that his experience at the asylum had convinced him that mental illness was more common in women (Dickens, 1856). This observation was just one of many, inherited from the Middle Ages and originating as far back as Hippocrates and Plato, which had led to the belief that mental illness was much more prevalent among women. Many explanations have been proposed. However, all revolved around the same idea: the ovaries, fallopian tubes and uterus were always held responsible, in varying order of importance.

At the time, although the function of these organs was still far from understood, experimental evidence indicated that they had much stronger interrelations than previously assumed. In 1775, Percival Pott reported that removal of both ovaries resulted in menstruation´s cessation in a young woman, giving rise to several theories attempting to explain the relationship between the ovaries and the uterus (O'Dowd & Philipp, 2000). Others had observed that women experienced physical and emotional changes each month, directly related to the menstrual cycles. Among them, Sir Henry Maudsley, a prominent physician of the era and pioneer of modern psychiatry in England, noted that *"the monthly activity of the ovaries has a marked effect on the body and mind and, therefore, may become a significant cause of physical and mental illness" (*Maudsley, 1884*)*. Thus, based on highly circumstantial experience, by the second half of the nineteenth century, the prevailing opinion held the ovaries responsible for the various symptoms and diseases associated with menstruation and the menstrual cycle. Disorders such as dysmenorrhea, chronic pelvic pain, and even vaguer conditions like hysteria were already being attributed to the ovaries, with various treatments proposed for their resolution (Chairou, 1870).

A. Sanabria and C. Betancourt, *Cognitive Biases in Surgical Practice*,
https://doi.org/10.1007/978-3-032-20377-9_22

Meanwhile, since McDowell's original experience in 1809 and following the introduction of anesthesia in 1846, oophorectomy had increasingly been performed to treat ovarian tumors. Soon, reports began to emerge of patients undergoing surgery for ovarian tumors who were also "*cured*" of other physical and mental ailments by the surgical intervention (Pozzi, 1905). In this context, the figure of Robert Battey would emerge with his revolutionary treatment.

Battey (Fig. 22.1) was born in Rome, Georgia in 1828. He studied medicine and later obstetrics in Philadelphia, earning his specialist degree in 1857. After graduation, as was customary among physicians from wealthy families, he traveled to Europe to visit leading medical centers, especially in England, where he had the opportunity to meet Spencer Wells, the most renowned ovarian surgeon of the time. Upon returning to the United States, with the outbreak of the American Civil War, he served for five years in the Confederate Army, operating on hundreds of severely wounded soldiers. After the war, he returned to his hometown, where he began a private practice dedicated to women's health. A serious, academic, well-connected man, deeply concerned for his patients, he quickly established a successful and growing clinical practice, which enabled him to become Professor of Gynecology and Obstetrics at the Atlanta Medical College. He also became editor-in-chief of the Atlanta Journal of Medicine and Surgery, founded the Georgia Gynecological Society and helped establish the American Gynecological Society (Thiery, 1998).

By 1870, at just 42 years old, he was one of the most recognized and respected gynecologists in the United States. In the middle of that year, a colleague asked him to evaluate his wife, who had gained an excessive amount of weight in recent months. For Battey, it was clear that this was a massive ovarian tumor, contrary to what other colleagues had considered to be obesity. Due to his training and experience, he knew that these tumors, although usually benign, could grow large enough to become fatal. After extensive analysis, he decided to operate on the woman. The surgery, which

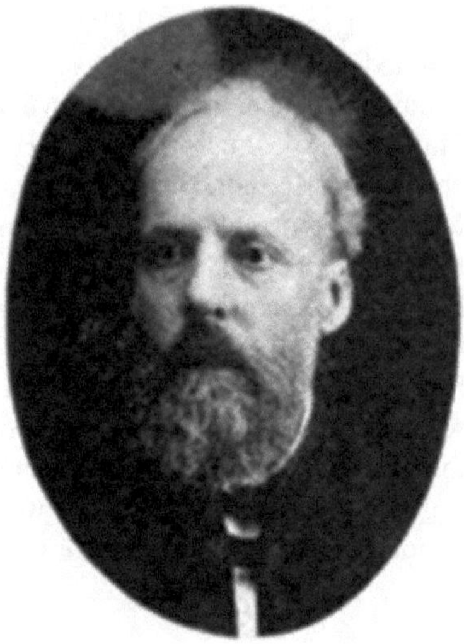

Fig. 22.1 Dr. Robert Battey (public domain). *Source* Unknown author

involved the removal of one ovary, was a complete success, with a rapid return to normal figure and weight. Following this successful experience, he began to explore the field of oophorectomy for clear gynecological conditions, always tumors. In 1872, however, this began to change.

During his years of clinical practice, Battey had encountered several patients with cyclical physical and psychological disorders that seemed related to menstruation but lacked clear explanations that could suggest a form of treatment. Among these, a woman named Mary would change him forever. Only 21 years old and of extraordinary beauty, she was first evaluated by Battey in 1865. For five years, she had suffered from severe monthly vascular and nervous disturbances, never having menstruated. Monthly episodes of endocarditis began to threaten her life. After a thorough physical examination, Battey found it evident that the woman had no uterus, which was undoubtedly the source of all her problems. According to the beliefs of the time, the ovaries produced a significant physiological alteration each month, which the body expelled through menstruation. If a woman had no uterus, the body could not rid itself of this alteration, which gave rise to all her ailments. If only there were a way to pacify the ovaries, Mary would be cured of all her health problems. The idea of oophorectomy crossed his mind; however, after many consultations and deliberations, Battey discovered that such a proposal was unprecedented and had not been previously considered by anyone. He himself had no experience with the procedure. Thus, month after month, he watched as Mary's health deteriorated further until her eventual death from heart failure. The autopsy confirmed his diagnosis: indeed, the woman had no uterus. Amid the grief and frustration of not having been able to help his patient, Battey promised himself that he would never let this happen again. He would not allow another woman to die without having tried to help her (Battey, 1887). In 1872, the opportunity would arise to put his revolutionary ideas into practice.

At just 23 years old, Julia had suffered for six years from monthly episodes of abdominal pain, rectal bleeding, discoloration of the abdominal wall, and "*rheumatism*" (a neurological syndrome with seizures and altered consciousness) that had been associated with cough in the past year. During this same period, she had menstruated only twice, had been hospitalized three times for intra-abdominal abscesses diagnosed as corporeal endometriosis, and had received treatment with silver nitrate, achieving only partial improvement. After a fourth abdominal abscess that spontaneously drained through the rectum, she was evaluated by Battey, who was already familiar with her case and had participated in her treatment. This time, with the memory of Mary still vivid, Battey thought that if the ovaries were removed, Julia would recover from her ailments, and he proposed the surgical option to the patient, who immediately accepted, as "*her life was that of a living dead*" (Battey, 1887). In addition, Battey sought the consent of all her family members. On August 17, 1872, a procedure was performed in which both ovaries, which appeared normal, were removed. After a month of hospitalization and overcoming a bout of peritonitis, the patient was discharged. The symptoms had miraculously disappeared; there were no more pains, abscesses, or "*rheumatism*," and Julia's life returned to that of a "*normal*" woman. At the end of September, Battey published his experience in the Atlanta Journal of Medicine and Surgery, coining the term "*normal ovariotomy*" and proposing it as a treatment option for women with similar conditions. He also sent a letter to the Boston Gynecological Society requesting that the surgery be officially recommended for the management of these diseases. The Society's response was ambiguous, neither supporting nor opposing the procedure, leaving the decision to the judgment of the "*skilled, careful, and observant practicing physician*" (Westmoreland, 1873). For Battey, however, there was little doubt, and he immediately adopted the procedure as the first-line treatment for women with these conditions. By 1878, he had operated on 14 patients with similar problems and had two deaths. Due to its apparent success, from that year onward he began to progressively expand the indications for the surgery to include all kinds of conditions, from ovarialgia (chronic pelvic pain) and nymphomania to hystero-epilepsy (hysteria), moral insanity, and any mental illness that could be associated with menstrual cycles (Jarrell & Stahnisch, 2021). His publications had a significant impact, and hundreds of surgeons in the United States and around the world began to replicate his experience. Battey achieved worldwide fame, and the removal of normal ovaries became known as Battey's operation. By the early 1880s, normal ovariotomy had become one of the most frequently performed surgical procedures, with many surgeons expanding Battey's indications to include any type of mental illness. It is estimated that more than 150,000 women ultimately underwent the procedure (Van De Warker, 1906).

The unfortunate consequences of the procedure were not long in coming. Premature menopause and postoperative mortality were only part of the problem. With an ever-increasing number of indications, soon it became evident that surgery was not effective for all the conditions it was supposed to improve. Battey himself, at the height of the procedure in 1881, during the London Medical Congress, reported a mortality rate of 18%, with an effectiveness that, while close to 100% for diseases such as oophoro-epilepsy, dropped to around 50% for oophoralgia and was almost nil for oophoromania (Battey, 1881). Despite this, the procedure continued to be performed more frequently, and Battey himself even carried it out to treat conditions as absurd as melancholia in two patients. Years later, he stated about these patients that, although one had not done well, the other remained "*reasonably well so far.*" (Jarrell & Stahnisch, 2021) The abuse of the procedure, its risks and consequences, the questionable results, and the gradual realization that the ovaries were highly valuable organs for women led to a shift in perspective and the beginning of the decline of routine ovariotomy. By the annual meeting of the American Gynecological Society in 1885, many began to speak out, if not against the procedure itself, at least against the unnecessary castration of women with mental disorders. The following year, the renowned Sir Thomas Spencer Wells, president of the Royal College of Surgeons of England and personal surgeon to Queen Victoria, delivered a lecture entitled "*Castration of Women for Mental Disease*," giving the final blow to the procedure by stating that "*its use for mental diseases is, to put it simply, unjustifiable.*" Two years later, the surgery was formally condemned by the American Gynecological Society (Thiery, 1998). Despite this, Battey continued to defend the procedure until the end of his days, stating that it "*will always have a place in the treatment of certain physical as well as mental conditions*" (Battey, 1887).

The story of Battey is a sad example of how someone can cause harm, despite having the best intentions and motivations and a solid background. What happened? While the initial idea was logical according to the knowledge of the time and the first results were apparently satisfactory, why continue with the procedure when the outcomes began to fall short? Why broaden the indications further when it was already clear that it was not effective for most conditions for which it was being used? And all this without mention the sequelae of the surgery and the high mortality rate, which was completely unacceptable considering that it was being used to treat benign diseases, mostly mental, that did not endanger the patients' lives. Was Battey a madman who simply wanted to mutilate women? Clearly not. Was he unaware of what he was doing or proposing? Neither. Was he ignorant of the results of his procedures? No, in his own letters and presentations, it was clear what was happening. So, what happened? The answer probably lies in one of the most dangerous cognitive biases when making analyses and estimates: survivorship bias.

Definition

Survivor bias is the flawed cognitive process by which, when conducting an analysis or estimation, only those results that have passed or "*survived*" a given selective process are considered, ignoring all the rest that did not. Thus, a "*successful*" subgroup is considered to represent the entire group, which renders all conclusions drawn from this analysis incorrect, as the information considered is incomplete and inaccurate. By considering only a portion of the total population, survivorship bias is a form of statistical selection bias, which usually leads to overly optimistic or positive estimates, since negative results, the "*non-survivors*" or unsuccessful cases, are typically left out of consideration.

In Battey's story, we see how he consistently focused on highlighting the positive outcomes of his interventions, the patients who had improved or been cured of their health problems. Even as the years went by and more and more patients failed to improve, suffered the consequences of premature menopause, or worse, died during surgery (outcomes known to him), Battey continued to insist not only on performing the surgery but also on expanding its indications because there were patients who improved, who were "*successful.*" Clearly, by focusing only on this subgroup of patients and ignoring the less fortunate, Battey had a distortedly positive view of the situation, considering his surgery to be useful, valuable, and even necessary for these patients.

History

The term survivor bias emerged after the work of Abraham Wald during World War II (Group, 1943; Wallis, 1980). At the time, Wald, a professor of statistics at Columbia University, had been assigned to the Statistical Research Group at the U.S. Navy Analysis Center. His mission was to conduct rigorous scientific analyses to generate strategies that could impact on the war. Faced with the question of where the fuselage of airplanes should be reinforced, the Group had conducted a series of analyses on planes returning from battle, determining the locations where bullets had struck. According to the diagrams, the answer seemed quite obvious: reinforcement should be applied to the wings and tail of the aircraft. However, Wald strongly opposed this initial analysis. His reasoning was truly clear: the planes that returned were only a portion of the population that should be analyzed, they were the "*survivors*," since despite the damage, they were able to return to base after battle. The other planes, the "*non-survivors*," those that did not return to base and were not included in the initial analysis, were the ones of real interest, as these suffered catastrophic damage that caused the aircraft to be lost. Thus, the part that needed to be reinforced was not the wings and tail, but rather the engine, since the diagrams showed no damage in this area, which was equivalent to saying that planes with bullet impacts in this zone crashed and did not return to base.

Subsequent studies expanded Wald's initial conclusions and extended their impact to all areas of human knowledge. Analyses and estimations in finance, social phenomena, historical studies, trading, marketing, health, investments, psychology, etc.; nothing escapes the influence of this bias. Of particular importance are the works of Kahneman and Tversky (Kahneman, 2011), who laid the foundations for understanding why this bias occurs, demonstrating that the human brain tends to consider only what it can see or what it deems important.

Impact

Given its presence in every facet of human life, survivor bias can negatively affect outcomes in multiple ways. Among the most significant are:

At the Personal Level:

1. **Misrepresentations of reality:** By causing the brain to focus only on a subset of the total population, the perception of the situation or problem under analysis will always be flawed, and any conclusions drawn from it will be fundamentally incorrect. Battey's story is an unfortunate example of this.
2. **Overestimation of success rates:** By paying attention only to positive or successful cases, the likelihood of success or effectiveness of any attempt, intervention, or strategy is systematically overestimated, which in turn creates a false sense of confidence.

3. **Underestimation of risks and failures:** By excluding negative cases, the bias masks risks, challenges, or potential vulnerabilities that may prove crucial and decisive when making decisions and planning any attempt or intervention.
4. **Negative impact on decision-making:** By creating a distorted image of reality, the resulting conclusions are erroneous. Any decision made based on this information will lead to the development of suboptimal strategies with unsatisfactory outcomes.

At the Collective Level:

1. **Faulty generalizations:** By focusing only on successful cases, bias can lead to incorrect generalized conclusions about trends, patterns, and even causal relationships. When findings are generalized based on biased information, vital details, problems, and difficulties that only failed cases can reveal are overlooked.
2. **Confusing correlation with causation:** By examining only the success stories of a particular behavior, strategy, or intervention, patterns (correlations) may be observed that can mislead and provide a false sense of causality. These erroneous patterns, by not considering all those who followed the same path but were unsuccessful, can lead to the adoption of behaviors and interventions that have no real connection to the perceived success.
3. **Creation of historical narratives:** It has often been said that "*history is written by the victors*," which is simply another manifestation of survivor bias. Only the individuals or groups who survived a battle, disease, problematic situation, calamity, conflict, etc., can write about it, conveying their experiences and opinions. These represent only a partial view of the event, as the experiences and perspectives of those who did not survive are equally important for a complete, objective, and impartial understanding of what occurred. Unfortunately, these are never written down or preserved. Therefore, most historical narratives upon which visions, ideals, trends, and behaviors are built are nothing more than incomplete fragments of past events, and this should be considered when establishing future lessons.

Examples in Medical and Surgical Practice

As we have noted, survivor bias affects every facet of human knowledge. The practice of medicine and surgery is no exception. Among its most significant effects, we can cite:

1. **Overestimation of favorable medium- and long-term outcomes:** Whether evaluating survival rates for a particular type of cancer after treatment, the long-term success of a procedure, or the probability of surviving trauma, excluding a portion of the population from analysis will systematically yield results that are better than the actual figures. For example, overestimating the probability of surviving a pulmonary trauma by evaluating only patients who made it to the hospital, while ignoring those who died before receiving care.

2. **Overestimation of chances of success:** By considering only the positive outcomes of a particular treatment or surgery, the apparent chances of success will be higher than they are. For example, the initial results of radical mastectomy in the early twentieth century for breast cancer only reflected the outcomes of survivors, without accounting for the women who died.
3. **Underestimation of risks or complications:** Another consequence of considering only positive outcomes is that the drawbacks related to a particular procedure or treatment will be systematically ignored and considered less frequent and/or less important than they are. For example, the excessive recommendation of major surgical procedures by only presenting patients who survive them, without considering all those who die or suffer severe complications.
4. **Generalization of practices based on studies conducted in selected populations:** Of relevance in diseases classified by stages such as cancer, this often leads to the generalization of a specific treatment strategy for each stage. However, if the studies that led to such conclusions did not include the entire patient population for specific reasons (inclusion or exclusion criteria, etc.), the generalization is incorrect because the results only apply to the patients who were considered. For example, considering surgery as the best option for all patients at a certain stage of a particular cancer when the studies only included patients who were eligible for surgery (comorbidities, extent of surgery, reconstruction possibilities, etc.).

How to Avoid Falling into Bias

1. **Examine all available data:** When evaluating any procedure, treatment, or situation, ensure that the entire population is assessed and that the data obtained represents all outcomes and experiences, no matter how unlikely they may seem. Likewise, use appropriate, comprehensive, diverse, and unbiased data sources. Always consider what might be missing.
2. **Use appropriate statistical analysis techniques:** Tools such as regression models, survival analysis, or propensity score matching have been developed to reduce the impact of survivor bias in statistical analyses. Understanding how these work and when to apply each is essential to avoid drawing erroneous conclusions.
3. **Actively look for third-party opinions:** Systematically include individuals with different perspectives when conducting analyses or attempting to draw conclusions about any procedure, strategy, or situation. Their insights and feedback will enrich any analysis, broaden the range of scenarios considered, strengthen the credibility and reliability of the conclusions, and mitigate the potential effects of bias.
4. **Recognize that errors are also a source of learning:** Beyond the natural disappointment of not achieving the desired outcome, failures are an invaluable source of growth. Instead of discarding, hiding, or forgetting them, learn to use them

as opportunities for improvement. Keeping them in mind during analysis, and fostering this culture within the team, helps mitigate the effects of bias.

5. **Systematically question the conclusions reached:** Regardless of how confident you are about a treatment, procedure, or situation, its frequency, or its likelihood of success, routinely consider the possibility that you may be mistaken and seek new arguments that could support this presumption. This will force you to consider other scenarios, populations, or possibilities that may have been excluded from the initial analysis and led to erroneous conclusions. In meetings or group discussions, proactively assign individuals to challenge the group consensus, no matter how uncomfortable or far-fetched their opinions may seem.

References

Battey, R. (1881). Oophorectomy–Battey's operation–Spaying-castration of women. Transactions of the International Medical Congress.

Battey, R. (1887). A history of Battey's operation: A review of the early history of normal ovariotomy-The difficulties encountered-professional Brethren Holding nightly caucuses awaiting the death of the first patient in order to arrest the operator-their disappointment-advice from friends-opposition from Medical journals-his first recognition by the profession-It comes from the literary hub-hope dawning-the present aspects of the operation-its future-advice to young doctors, Etc. An address delivered before the atlanta society of medicine, December 3, 1886. *Atlanta Med Surg J (1884)*, *3*(11), 657–675.

Chairou, É. (1870). *Études cliniques sur l'hystérie, nature, lésions anatomiques, traitement*. Baillière. https://books.google.com.co/books?id=O7ZYAAAAcAAJ

Dickens, C. (1856). *Household words /conducted by Charles Dickens*. B. Tauchnitz. https://books.google.com.co/books?id=rKrJzgEACAAJ

Group, C. U. S. R. (1943). *A method of estimating plane vulnerability based on damage of survivors: An equation satisfied by the probabilities that a plane will be downed by 1 hits*. Applied Mathematics Panel, National Defense Research Committee. https://books.google.com.co/books?id=hZtWtAEACAAJ

Jarrell, J., & Stahnisch, F. W. (2021). Contextualizing ovarian pain in the late 19th century—Part 2: Ovarian-based treatments of "hysteria." *Journal of the History of the Neurosciences, 30*(4), 375–389. https://doi.org/10.1080/0964704X.2021.1902065

Kahneman, D. (2011). *Thinking, fast and slow*. Farrar, Straus and Giroux. https://books.google.com.co/books?id=ZuKTvERuPG8C

Maudsley, H. (1884). *Sex in mind and in education*. C.W. Bardeen. https://books.google.com.co/books?id=T19Jjndz7qEC

O'Dowd, M. J., & Philipp, E. E. (2000). *The history of obstetrics & gynaecology*. CRC Press. https://books.google.com.co/books?id=qS0QyAEACAAJ

Pozzi, S. (1905). *Traité de gynécologie clinique et opératoire*. Masson. https://wellcomecollection.org/works/f29fa9ge/items

Thiery, M. (1998). Battey's operation: An exercise in surgical frustration. *European Journal of Obstetrics, Gynecology, and Reproductive Biology, 81*(2), 243–246. https://doi.org/10.1016/s0301-2115(98)00197-3

Van De Warker, E. (1906). The fetich of the ovary. *American Journal of Obstetrics and Diseases of Women and Children, 54*, 366–373.

Wallis, W. A. (1980). The statistical research group, 1942–1945. *Journal of the American Statistical Association, 75*(370), 320–330. https://doi.org/10.2307/2287451

Westmoreland, W. F. (1873). Editorial correspondence. *Atlanta Med Surg J, 10*(10), 616–618.

Chapter 23
Illusion of Control: The Fastest Knife in the West End

The Problem

A good surgeon must possess many qualities: fine manual dexterity, meticulousness, attention to detail, precision, composure and detailed anatomical knowledge are indispensable and unquestionable. Others, such as adaptability, physical and mental endurance, nonlinear thinking, emotional stability, teamwork, desire for continuous learning, leadership, and empathy are important, though not strictly essential. However, no quality generates as much confusion, astonishment, and controversy as speed. Often regarded as a measure of skill, the two terms are frequently used interchangeably. Yet, whether this is truly the case is debatable. This raises the question of whether a surgeon presumed to be skilled is always fast, whether a good surgeon must be fast, or whether speed is a defining and indispensable quality for excellence in surgery.

History is full of examples of great surgical figures who were not known for their speed. Conversely, there are many others who are remembered and even celebrated for their extreme velocity in performing operations. Among the latter, perhaps none is more famous than Dr. Robert Liston, a Scottish surgeon of the Victorian era. In a time when anesthesia did not exist yet and the principles of asepsis and antisepsis were entirely unknown, speed in surgery was an invaluable asset and often made the difference between successfully completing a procedure or witnessing a patient flee the operating room in terror. In this context, the iconic figure of Liston emerged, who would be nicknamed and remembered for posterity as *"the fastest knife in the West End" (Wright & Maxwell,* 2014*).*

Robert Liston (Fig. 23.1) was born on October 28, 1794, in West Lothian, a small town in Scotland. The son of a Catholic reverend, his mother died when he was only six years old, leaving his early education entirely in his father´s hands. At just 14, he entered the University of Edinburgh, and two years later began his studies in medicine and surgery under the renowned anatomist John Barclay (Magee, 1999).

A. Sanabria and C. Betancourt, *Cognitive Biases in Surgical Practice*,
https://doi.org/10.1007/978-3-032-20377-9_23

Four years later, he was admitted as a house surgeon at the Royal Infirmary of Edinburgh, and two years later, at only 22, he was recognized as a surgeon by the Royal College of Surgeons of London (Mian et al., 2013). He began his professional practice at the same Royal Infirmary of Edinburgh, where he quickly gained a reputation as an intimidating and argumentative surgeon, highly demanding of his assistants and students and with extraordinarily little tolerance for error. At the same time, he developed a unique surgical practice, focusing primarily on treating patients who had not been admitted to the Royal Infirmary because they were considered unfit for surgery due to severe conditions or illnesses. This eventually led to conflicts with his surgical colleagues, whom he criticized, and with the Infirmary authorities, as the situation could be interpreted as Liston diverting patients from the institution for his own benefit (Wright & Maxwell, 2014). These circumstances led to ongoing disputes with the Infirmary, resulting in several temporary suspensions and his eventual departure in 1835, when he accepted the position of Professor of Clinical Surgery at the newly founded University College Hospital in London (Magee, 1999). He would remain there for the rest of his professional life.

Deeply concerned about the traumatic nature of surgical procedures for patients, he dedicated himself to perfecting and shortening them, especially amputations, which were the most common surgeries of his time. To this end, he modified the surgical techniques of the era and developed a series of instruments for these procedures, some of which are still in use today (Liston, 1838). All of this, combined with tremendous strength and exceptional skill, enabled him to routinely perform an amputation in under one minute, and on occasions in as little as 30s, figures of which Liston was especially proud (Hollingham, 2024). His fame spread rapidly, and soon surgeons from all over Great Britain and Europe filled his surgical theater to witness and learn his refined technique. This only further increased Liston's confidence and ego, who, like a showman, once the patient was ready and his gloves were on, would make it a habit to say to the audience *"Time me, gentlemen, time me!"* (Magee, 1999).

Beyond the spectacle, Liston's results were far superior to those of his peers. Between 1835 and 1840 alone, he performed 66 amputations with only 10 deaths, a mortality rate of 1 in 6. The best surgeons in London at the time had a mortality rate of 1 in 4 (Thomas, 2012).

Beyond the speed of his procedures, these results were most likely explained by three factors rarely mentioned by Liston: First, in an era when the existence of germs and microorganisms was completely unknown and surgeons in practice were closer to butchers than to clinical physicians, Liston was extremely meticulous and demanding about hygiene and cleanliness. He routinely washed his hands at the beginning and end of each surgery and required his assistants to thoroughly clean the instruments after every procedure. He also wore a clean gown for each new operation, contrary to the custom of wearing the same gown throughout the surgical day, regardless of whether it was covered in blood, pus, or any other type of secretion (Hollingham, 2024). Second, Liston was a profound expert in anatomy, which in his view was the most important quality any surgeon should possess (Liston, 1838). This knowledge not only gave him confidence and speed but also allowed him to avoid serious accidents during his operations, as he knew in detail where to find each vital

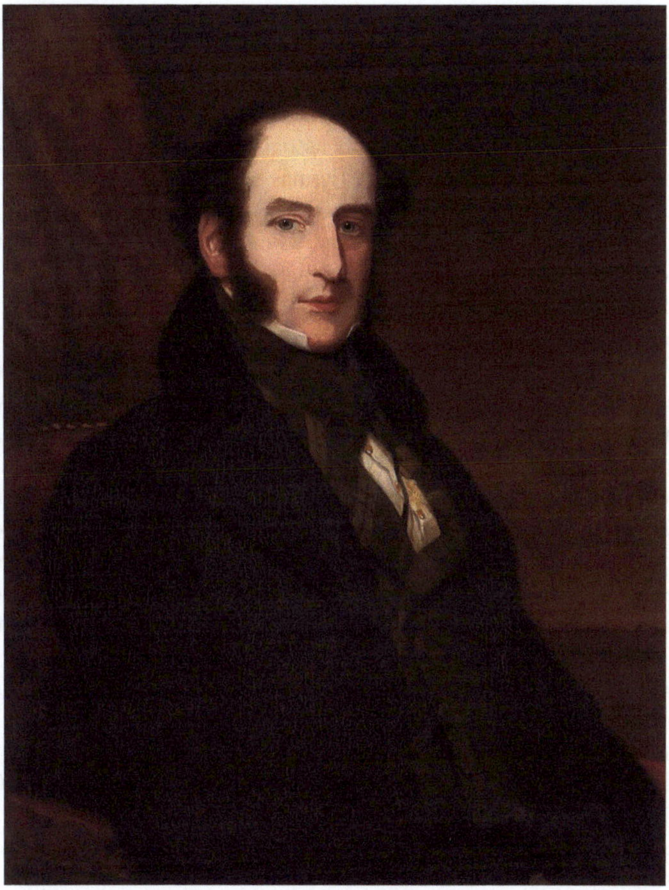

Fig. 23.1 Robert Liston (public domain). *Source* Samuel John Stump—Art UK

structure. Third, Liston is probably the first surgeon in history to formally recognize the importance of postoperative care. As he noted in his treatises, a surgeon's work only begins once the surgery is over (Liston, 2022). Thus, contrary to the custom of the time, he placed much more importance on postoperative care than on the surgery itself, following and monitoring his patients until they were able to leave the hospital. Despite all his successes, his constant obsession with speed was not without unfortunate incidents.

There are at least two infamous incidents associated with Liston, both occurring during amputations and clearly explained by his preoccupation with speed. In one case, in his enthusiasm, he amputated not only the patient's leg but also his testicles. The second incident, known as the only surgery with a 300% mortality rate, is the most enduring episode in Liston's history, despite all his previously mentioned achievements. During this procedure, in his rush for speed, he amputated not only the patient's leg but also the fingers of one of his assistants who was helping to hold the patient steady. Both later died because of infectious complications. Additionally, at some point during the operation, the scalpel flew out of his hand toward the audience, tearing the coat of one of the spectators. Believing he had been seriously injured, the man fainted and later died from injuries sustained due to fall. Thus, for the only time in history, a single surgical procedure was associated with three deaths: the patient, the surgeon's assistant and a bystander (Thomas, 2012).

Without a doubt, Liston, with his successes and missteps, is one of the most emblematic figures of Victorian-era surgery, with many characteristics that define a good surgeon: meticulousness, skill, determination, detailed anatomical knowledge, high standards, attention to detail, deep concern for the patient, ingenuity, capacity for innovation, and so on. But, returning to the initial question, what can be said about his speed? In Liston's time, surgeons had to be fast, but it is not known whether this trait made surgeons better, or if a fast surgeon was, in fact, a better one. Liston, who more than anyone before or since has embodied speed in a surgeon, can help find the answer. During a lecture to his students at University College London in 1844, Liston said, "*You must study to perform surgery with the least possible pain for the patient, and to do that you must be as quick as possible...*" (Liston, 1846). This sounds a bit far-fetched, even for someone as colorful as Liston. While it can be said that quick surgery might reduce the duration of a painful experience in an era when anesthesia did not exist, the intensity of the unpleasant subjective sensation defined as pain is exactly the same, regardless of how long a procedure lasts. Even today, with procedures routinely performed under anesthesia, pain remains an unwanted companion of every postoperative period.

So, what was going on with Liston? Was he justifying his mistakes with this argument? Was he, driven by his ego, convinced he could eliminate pain? Or did he sincerely believe what he said, and his motivation was simply to help his patients? The answer probably lies in the illusion of control, one of the most observed cognitive biases in surgery.

Definition

The illusion of control is defined as a probabilistic expectation of success that is inappropriately higher than what objective probability would suggest (Langer, 1975). In other words, the illusion of control is the tendency to overestimate the degree of control one has over the outcome of uncontrollable events or those determined primarily by chance.

In life, there are two major elements that determine the satisfactory outcome of any activity or task: the capacity or skill to perform the work and chance or luck. In turn, there are events determined entirely by chance, such as lottery results, gambling, etc., and other events where skill plays a predominant role, such as performing surgery, interpreting a piano piece, etc. The illusion of control arises when these scenarios are confused, and one believes it is possible to exert control over chance. Experimental evidence has shown that this bias appears when elements typical of skill-based events are mixed with scenarios where luck is the main determinant (Langer, 1975) (Alloy & Abramson, 1979). Among these elements, the most studied are familiarity with the task, active involvement, previous success, clarity of the desired outcome, mood, and need for control.

In Liston's story, the magnitude of a person's painful experience is fundamentally determined by the intensity of the painful stimulus and the patient's pain threshold. If the painful stimulus was always the same (amputation), the magnitude of the painful experience was determined by the patient's pain threshold. Based on current knowledge, it is impossible to exert control over this element, so we can say it is determined by chance. Thus, neither Liston nor anyone else can control the pain threshold. However, when elements such as familiarity with the task (amputations were the most frequently performed surgery by Liston, in which he was considered an expert), clarity of the desired outcome (amputations with the least possible pain), and especially very active involvement in the task (precise, efficient, and above all, very rapid amputations) are introduced, the illusion of control appears, with Liston believing that by being very fast he would be able to reduce the magnitude of the pain.

History

The term illusion of control was coined by Ellen Langer, a psychologist at Yale University, in 1975 (Langer, 1975). In her initial publication, Langer presented six experiments constructed in scenarios entirely governed by chance. In each of these, the introduction of some elements commonly associated with controllable events, mainly skill, led participants to overestimate their ability to control uncontrollable events that depended entirely on chance. Subsequent experiments, in different scenarios and situations, have confirmed Langer's initial observations. Among these, the work of Thompson is particularly noteworthy (Thompson et al., 1998). He introduced the term control heuristic to explain why the bias arises. In his publication, he notes that the bias is produced by the combination of two factors: the desire to achieve the set goal and the presence of apparent (not real) connections between the action and the desired outcome. Later, to further expand on the dangerous consequences of the bias, Kahneman established that, while there are activities entirely determined by chance, there are no activities entirely governed by skill, because even in these, chance is always present to a greater or lesser degree, playing a decisive role in achieving the desired outcome (Kahneman, 2011).

Impact

The illusion of control can affect people in a wide variety of contexts and situations, encompassing all aspects of life. Among the most important are:

At the Personal Level:

1. **Incorrect risk assessment:** When the ability to control situations and achieve desired goals is overestimated, a false sense of security and excessive optimism is created. This leads to a distorted assessment of the risk faced in each scenario, as one believes to be more capable or to have control over situations that are, by their nature, completely uncontrollable.
2. **Poor decision-making:** Because of the previous point, the decisions made to address each situation will always fall short of being ideal. Thus, with the overconfidence that accompanies the overestimation of abilities, there is a tendency to design or choose strategies that are simpler and easier than the situation requires, with less preparation, effort, and study than is necessary.
3. **Adoption of rituals and/or habits:** Believing that one can influence actions over which there is no control leads to the establishment of incoherent and even laughable causal relationships that determine decisions, habits, and life practices. Thus, for example, if on the day a new pair of shoes is worn for the first time an accident occurs on the way to work, it is assumed that those new shoes are "*bad luck*" and they are not worn again. As absurd as it may seem, society is full of students wearing their "*lucky socks*" every time they take an exam, athletes who do not shave when playing crucial matches, or fans who, when going to watch their team, wear the same cap or shirt.
4. **Gambling and betting addiction:** Betting, lotteries, casino games, and other similar activities are entirely controlled by chance. However, there are people deeply involved in them despite constant losses. This is because they believe that with enough study and dedication, they will be able to decipher or control the outcome, which is impossible.

At the Collective Level:

1. **Belief in magical and/or paranormal:** Rare and unlikely events occur under the total and absolute responsibility of chance. However, instead of accepting them as such, anomalies statistics, human beings search for plausible explanations in which individuals have had or may exert some type of influence, thus ending up believing in miracles, energies, paranormal phenomena, the power of will, etc., in an attempt to explain these events. When this way of thinking is passed down from generation to generation, magical traditions, myths, legends, and customs are acquired, which characterize each society.

Examples in Medical and Surgical Practice

The practice of medicine and surgery involves constant decision-making and the execution of actions aimed at assessing and improving patients' health status. Sadly, it is impossible for this to be exempt from the effects of the illusion of control. Among the most important examples are:

1. **Overdiagnosis:** Ordering unnecessary or irrelevant tests based on the condition or stage of the disease being evaluated, to ensure a better outcome. For example, ordering preoperative tests for a healthy adolescent or requesting a PET-CT scan to rule out metastatic disease in an early-stage thyroid cancer.
2. **Overtreatment:** Also known as "*therapeutic illusion*," this occurs when unnecessary medications are prescribed to treat self-limiting diseases or to prevent complications that do not warrant such intervention. It also includes unnecessarily increasing the extent of surgeries in a futile attempt to improve the patient's prognosis. For example, using hemostatic agents in surgeries with minimal bleeding risk, such as a cholecystectomy, or performing radical prostatectomies in cases of low-risk prostate tumors.
3. **Estimation of surgical risk or life expectancy prognosis:** Believing that one has control over uncontrollable factors leads to completely erroneous assessments. The risks of various surgical procedures are underestimated, and the prognosis of diseases is either improved or worsened depending on how early or advanced they may appear. For example, the surgeon who assures the patient that "*everything will go perfectly*" because "I *am the one operating,*" ignoring that there may be factors beyond their surgical skill that influence the outcome; or the oncologic surgeon who tells the patient they have "*one month to live*" because their cancer is very advanced.
4. **Indication of highly aggressive and radical surgeries in advanced cancer stages** when the patient's prognosis is determined by factors beyond the reach of surgery, such as the biological behavior of the tumor, the patient's immune status, etc., which cannot be influenced by a surgical procedure. For example, Halsted radical mastectomies that could involve resecting the rib cage, which made no difference in prognosis.
5. **Surgical rituals and customs:** The illusion of control can lead to the establishment of absurd, incoherent, and even laughable associations and causal relationships. For example, the surgeon who always operates on difficult cases wearing the same surgical cap because it brings good luck, or who believes that the outcome of the surgery depends on the music playing in the operating room.

How to Avoid Falling into This Bias?

1. **Learn about and understand the illusion of control:** As with all cognitive biases, being aware of its existence, scope, and implications is an essential step to avoid falling into it. Understanding that some situations depend on skill and others on chance, how these can become intertwined, how to differentiate them, and the factors that facilitate confusion between the two (familiarity, involvement, previous successes, etc.) is of utmost importance.
2. **Make intentional and realistic assessments of control:** In every new situation or decision to be made, take a few minutes to objectively evaluate those aspects over which you have control and those that are completely beyond your reach.

Once this exercise is completed and your available capabilities are defined, you can make a more informed decision.

3. **Promote reflective thinking:** This involves actively and continuously questioning beliefs and assumptions about the environment in which we live and the control we can exert over it. Constantly doubting one's convictions helps mitigate the sense of control over situations. Strategies such as keeping a journal to record each decision made, the expected outcome at the time, and the actual result obtained, help to gauge the real control we have over the situations we face.
4. **Encourage group decision-making:** In the workplace, financial, and even family settings, involve as many people as possible in the decision-making process. Different viewpoints, especially those contraries to one's own, will enrich discussions by challenging various perspectives and will mitigate the illusion of control for each participant, allowing for more accurate and realistic decisions.
5. **Know and use the scientific method:** Various statistical and epidemiological concepts such as correlation, causality, association, and probability are fundamental for understanding chance and the role it plays in daily life. Learning and acquiring tools that enable their application to daily life will allow for a better understanding of those aspects over which we have no control, thus avoiding the confusion that gives rise to bias.

References

Alloy, L. B., & Abramson, L. Y. (1979). Judgment of contingency in depressed and nondepressed students: Sadder but wiser? *Journal of Experimental Psychology: General, 108*(4), 441–485. https://doi.org/10.1037//0096-3445.108.4.441

Hollingham, R. (2024). *Blood and guts: A history of surgery*. Macmillan.

Kahneman, D. (2011). *Thinking, fast and slow*. Farrar, Straus and Giroux. https://books.google.com.co/books?id=ZuKTvERuPG8C

Langer, E. J. (1975). The illusion of control. *Journal of Personality and Social Psychology, 32*(2), 311–328. https://doi.org/10.1037/0022-3514.32.2.311

Liston, R. (1838). *Practical surgery: With one hundred and twenty engravings on wood*. James Crissy.

Liston, R. (1846). *Lectures on the operations of surgery: And on diseases and accidents requiring operations*. Lea and Blanchard.

Liston, R. (2022). *Elements of surgery*. DigiCat.

Magee, R. (1999). Robert Liston: Surgeon extraordinary. *Australian and New Zealand Journal of Surgery, 69*(12), 878–881. https://doi.org/10.1046/j.1440-1622.1999.01721.x

Mian, A., Shoja, M. M., Watanabe, K., Rozzelle, C. J., Loukas, M., & Tubbs, R. S. (2013). Robert Liston (1794–1847): Surgical anatomist and resurrectionist with an interest in hydrocephalus. *Childs Nervous System, 29*(1), 1–4. https://doi.org/10.1007/s00381-012-1994-3

Thomas, B. (2012). Saints and sinner: Robert Liston. *The Bulletin of the Royal College of Surgeons of England, 94*(2), 64–65. https://doi.org/10.1308/147363512x13189526439197

Thompson, S. C., Armstrong, W., & Thomas, C. (1998). Illusions of control, underestimations, and accuracy: A control heuristic explanation. *Psychological Bulletin, 123*(2), 143–161. https://doi.org/10.1037/0033-2909.123.2.143

Wright, A. S., & Maxwell, P. J. t. (2014). Robert Liston, M.D. (October 28, 1794-December 7, 1847): The fastest knife in the West End. *Am Surg, 80* (1), 1–2. https://www.ncbi.nlm.nih.gov/pubmed/24401493

Appendix

General and Specific Checklist to Prevent Cognitive Biases

General Checklist

Use before making a surgical decision, even in apparently routine scenarios,

☐ I acknowledge the possibility of bias and recalibrate my thinking.

☐ I take a brief pause (30–60 seconds) to slow down automatic thinking before determining a surgical course of action.

☐ I actively question my first impression or the group's automatic consensus.

☐ I look for objective, pertinent, and relevant information for the problem to be solved.

☐ I consider that I can choose to wait and obtain more information.

☐ I always consider other opinions.

☐ I use an applicable checklist, algorithm, or clinical scoring system.

☐ I document my reasoning: risks, benefits, and arguments supporting the decision.

Specific Checklists

1. **Causality (Etiology)**

These items are related to:

- Distinguishing correlation from causation
- Controlling for confounding
- Identifying whether "perceived" risks are real
- Eliminating irrelevant variables that distort causality

☐ I verify that my conclusion logically follows from the data, not from beliefs or intuition.

A. Sanabria and C. Betancourt, *Cognitive Biases in Surgical Practice*,
https://doi.org/10.1007/978-3-032-20377-9

☐ I distinguish correlation from causation and confirm that the proposed course of action has rational and scientific support.

☐ I identify whether I am reasoning under fear, haste, sympathy, frustration, or a desire to prove something, or if these factors unjustifiably amplify or minimize my judgment.

☐ I discard any anecdotal information (colleagues' stories, subjective experiences, informal claims) or information lacking direct clinical basis.

☐ I avoid being influenced by striking stories, rumors, or sensational news.

☐ I check whether my personal risk perception (risk-seeking or risk-averse) is biasing my judgment.

☐ I avoid reinterpreting the case considering previous outcomes.

☐ I check whether my negative view of a factor is affecting my assessment.

2. **Diagnosis**

These items are related to:

- Selecting information relevant to the case
- Making independent decisions for each clinical case
- Choosing clinical hypotheses protected from the influence of clinical hierarchies
- Using diagnostic tests rationally

☐ I review all relevant information: history, physical examination, imaging, laboratory results, and temporal evolution.

☐ I confirm that all data used are valid and up to date.

☐ I allocate more time for discussion and consideration to aspects with greater risk or uncertainty.

☐ I recognize that the decision is not based solely on prominent or readily available data.

☐ I use structured tools to assess information.

☐ I evaluate each idea on its clinical merit, not on the characteristics of the person presenting it.

☐ I ask: "Does anyone on the team see something I am missing?".

☐ I systematically look for information that challenges my opinions.

☐ I identify whether the possibility of a diagnostic error is leading me to perform unnecessary actions.

3. **Treatment (Therapeutics)**

These items are related to:

- Evaluating action versus inaction
- Justifying interventions
- Correctly choosing therapeutic alternatives
- Controlling hierarchical influence
- Avoiding false dilemmas
- Communicating risks and benefits
- Supervising technical quality

☐ I recognize that I am not as rational, skilled, capable, or precise as I believe myself to be.

☐ I avoid attributing to personal skill what is due to chance.

☐ I assess whether my decision to intervene or not intervene arises from prudence or from a desire to avoid responsibility.

☐ I compare the risks and benefits of acting versus not acting, and I include hybrid or conservative alternatives.

☐ I ask myself: "Do I agree out of clinical conviction, or due to deference, hierarchy, or team pressure?".

☐ I create space to question the plan before implementing it and ensure at least one dissenting perspective is included.

☐ I keep reasoning and discussion focused on criteria and data, not on affinities, personalities, or positions.

☐ I avoid phrases such as "we always do it this way" as the main justification.

☐ I exclude factors such as patient personality, administrative pressure, shift, team preferences, or historical routines.

4. **Prognosis**

These propositions are related to:

- Using prediction tools
- Analyzing the temporal relationship of the data
- Assessing long-term impact

☐ I assess whether the prognosis depends on my intervention, patient factors, or biological variability.

☐ I base my decisions on adjusted risk, probability of complications, survival models, or validated scores using prediction tools.

☐ I evaluate how the decision will affect the patient over weeks, months, and years, considering functional impact, quality of life, need for reintervention, and late sequelae.

☐ I broaden the time horizon of the prognostic analysis.

☐ I clarify concepts and correct misinformation with clear, up-to-date evidence.

☐ I define what I expect as a good outcome and the criteria for failure before deciding (safety, function, morbidity).

☐ I ensure traceability for audits and quality review.

☐ I review whether the way data are presented biases me toward a particular position.

Index

A. Sanabria and C. Betancourt, *Cognitive Biases in Surgical Practice*,
https://doi.org/10.1007/978-3-032-20377-9

MIX
Papier aus verantwortungsvollen Quellen
Paper from responsible sources
FSC® C105338

If you have any concerns about our products,
you can contact us on
ProductSafety@springernature.com

In case Publisher is established outside the EU,
the EU authorized representative is:
Springer Nature Customer Service Center GmbH
Europaplatz 3, 69115 Heidelberg, Germany

Printed by Libri Plureos GmbH
in Hamburg, Germany